Contents

About This

The Good News

Today's drugs are miraculous. They can halt infections, save lives, and turn what were once deadly conditions into minor problems. They can make life easier for those with chronic conditions and bring relief from pain and suffering. Millions of lives have been saved by antibiotics, insulin, high-blood pressure medications, and anti-cancer drugs.

The Bad News

Their great powers come with potential risks. If drugs are strong enough to help and heal, they are strong enough to harm as well. All medicines —prescription, over-the-counter, herbals—have side effects and can cause bad reactions. Some ill effects can't be predicted or prevented, but many can.

This Book Will Help You

- Get more out of doctor visits.
- Better utilize your pharmacist.
- Monitor side effects.
- Take your medications properly.
- Keep better records.
- Save money.
- Understand your medicines.

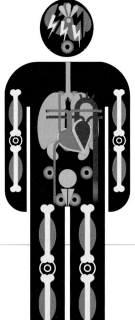

How We Did It

In compiling this book, we identified the prescription, over-the-counter, and herbal medications most commonly used to treat prevalent medical conditions and researched each using the sources most often used by doctors and pharmacists. Among them:

- The Federal Drug Administration
- Drug Facts and Comparisons (2000 edition)
- Handbook of Clinical Drug Data
- Hansten and Horn's Drug Interactions Analysis
- The Physicians' Drug Reference (PDR)
- PDR for Herbal Medicines
- The Pill Book

We discovered that the lists of possible side effects and interactions often differ between sources. So, we cross-referenced and listed those common to multiple sources, paring down the mountains of information into what would be most important to consumers.

Our most arduous task was crafting a way to present this information so that you can find in minutes what might take hours wading through professional medical texts. We created a format that allows you to quickly find the important side effects and interactions and easily compare common drugs used to treat a condition. Then we asked medical and pharmaceutical experts to review the text for accuracy.

Despite all of our efforts, though, it's important to remember that there is no universal or definitive source of medical information, for medicine is an art, as well as a science. Proving that a particular medicine causes a particular ill effect isn't always possible and medicines that help one person may harm another.

It is, therefore, all the more critical that you understand as much as you can about the medicines you take and develop a good working relationship with your doctors and pharmacist, especially if you take more than one medication. For in the end, it is up to you to know as much as you can about your most valuable asset, your health.

We hope you find this book a useful tool.

Body system indicators

Drugs in this book are organized by body system so you can read about all the alternatives for your treatment. In chapters 2 through 9, each body system is designated by a corresponding icon to assist in guiding you through the book.

Book

A question box appears in the upper righthand corner throughout chapter 1 and contains a question or thought that relates to information contained in the text on that particular page.

Alerts

You'll see this symbol next to certain drugs. This denotes that the drug has a narrow margin between the amount that can help you and the amount that will hurt you. These drugs must be dosed with extreme caution and monitored closely.

The drug banner

The name of each drug is contained within a color-coded bar. Drugs are listed alphabetically by their trade name with the generic name italicized in parentheses and the drug class following.

Drug banner color code:

Red banner: prescription

Blue banner: over-the-counter

Green banner: herbs

Price rating system

You'll see dollar signs next to the drug names. Prices range too much to report precise dollar amounts.

Following is the scale used:

Lowest cost	Highest cost
$ ——————————▶	$$$$$

(Below is a partial citation for colitis. Refer to the chapter on the Digestive System for the complete citation.)

Common drugs for colitis

Report any side effects to doctor if severe or persistent. Those in orange, report immediately.

Important side effects	Negative drug interactions	Special warnings
Asacol *(mesalamine)*, an anti-inflammatory		$$$$$
Abdominal cramps, diarrhea, dizziness, increased number of loose stools, appetite loss, headache, runny nose, sneezing, rash, itching, skin or eye discoloration, back or stomach pain, chills,...	*Do not combine with:* Benemid *(probenecid).* *Use caution with:* Azulfidine *(sulfasalazine)* and Coumadin *(warfarin).* Consult your doctor before combining these drugs with any other drug....	*Do not use if:* you have impaired kidney function; a sulfite or aspirin allergy; active ulcer disease; or have had a varicella vaccine in the past six weeks....

Important side effects

The first column lists the most common side effects and the dangerous side effects. Where the side effects are listed for a group of drugs, all drugs in the group may not have produced all side effects listed.

Negative drug interactions

The second column lists drugs that should not be taken together and drugs that can be combined only with caution.

Special warnings

The third column lists special warnings for older adults.

Drugs 101

How do drugs work?

prescription

over-the-counter

herbal

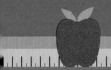

By better understanding your medications, you can reduce your risks and recognize problems at the earliest, least serious stages. You can help your doctors improve your care by keeping them informed about your symptoms.

Prescription Drugs

If you put a label on a bottle of water and claim that it treats dehydration, the **Food and Drug Administration** (FDA) considers it a drug and has the authority to regulate it. As long as you don't make any claim that a product has healing properties or will treat disease, the **FDA** doesn't consider it a drug and has no power to regulate.

Over-the-Counter (OTC) Medications

Generally less potent, these medications can be taken without a doctor's authorization. In large doses, though, OTC medications can exceed the strength of a prescription medication.

Herbal Supplements

Because herbs cannot be patented and regulated, distributors are not likely to devote the time and money necessary to prove that an herb is medically safe and efficacious. As a result, strength and quality vary wildly, making it difficult to know what the right dose is.

The expectation that you need a drug for every ache and pain is not realistic. You have to weigh benefits against risks.

Nutraceuticals

Nutraceuticals are food stuffs that have a pharmacological effect, which means they provide medical or health benefits, such as preventing or treating diseases. They might contain vitamins, minerals, or enzymes, and have healing properties, such as garlic, cayenne pepper, safflower oil. Benecol and Take Control, cholesterol-lowering margarines, are two examples.

How Drugs Are Taken

The 7 most common ways to deliver drugs:

- Oral (most popular)

- Transdermal (topical, e.g., estrogen patches)

- Intravenous (e.g., anesthetics)

- Intramuscular (vaccines)

- Subcutaneous (under the skin, e.g., insulin)

- Rectal (e.g., suppositories that treat colon inflammation)

- Inhalation (e.g., most asthma drugs)

Path of a Pill

After you swallow a pill or capsule, here are the four processes that take place:

Disintegration

First, the pill or capsule disintegrates in the stomach or small intestine.

Absorption

Next, the pill or capsule is absorbed. Most absorption takes place in the small intestine, although some acid-based drugs, like aspirin, start the absorption process in the stomach.

Distribution

Drugs enter the blood stream and pass through the liver, where enzymes can alter their potency. Reduced liver function means that more of the drug will circulate in the blood and remain effective. Then the drug enters the systemic circulation. It can enter cells, disperse in body water, or accumulate in organs, tissue, or body fat. It may bind to proteins in the blood or to tissue. It's only the portion of the drug that doesn't get bound that remains effective. Only a small percentage of some drugs get metabolized (or used). For example, only 1 to 3% of Coumadin doesn't bind to proteins.

Many drug problems suffered by older adults can be avoided or reversed if you provide complete and thorough information to your doctors and make sure you get information in return that will help you take medications correctly.

If you take any other drug that competes for protein, it could double the effect of the Coumadin.

Excretion

The part of the drug that isn't absorbed or distributed gets excreted, through saliva, sweat, respiration, breast milk, urine or feces. (The last two are the most common exits.) How rapidly drugs get excreted depends on output of the kidneys and liver. Thus, drugs stick around longer in those with reduced kidney or liver function. Liver and kidney function slowly decrease with age, so drug dosages are often reduced for older people.

How Drugs Work

Drugs basically act in the following four ways:

Drugs inhibit or block enzymes, receptors, or nerve impulses.

This is the most common form of action and includes pain-killing drugs like codeine, aspirin, and lidocaine.

Drugs stimulate nerve impulses.

They stimulate the nerves to transmit information over the network. This category includes stimulant drugs like epinephrine and antidepressants, such as Prozac.

Drugs work on living cells.

Antibiotics, for example, kill bacteria cells.

Drugs replace deficiencies.

Some drugs are taken to provide a substance in which your body is deficient, such as insulin, vitamins or hormones.

At the Doctor's Office

Many drug problems suffered by older adults can be avoided or reversed if you provide complete and thorough information to your doctors and make sure you get information in return that will help you take medications correctly.

Here's what you can do to get a lot more out of every visit to the doctor.

Don't Go Without These

There are four things you should always bring to the doctor:

- A list of your symptoms or problems and when they started.

Case Study

Sandra was a 58-year-old woman who developed blood clots in her leg, so her doctor prescribed Coumadin, a blood thinner. Several months after starting therapy, she was bothered by the hot flashes of menopause. She asked an employee of the health-food store what might help, and he suggested Dong Quai, which she began taking.

Sandra didn't tell her doctor about the Dong Quai, which contains coumarins, the therapeutic ingredient of Coumadin, (which itself is derived from clover). The combination effectively doubled the dose and overly thinned her blood and contributed to a complication of internal bleeding. Now she reports anything that might have a therapeutic effect—including vitamins, herbs, hormone supplements, and even herbal teas.

- Your pill profile or a bag with all the drugs you are taking—including prescription, over-the-counter, herbs, and herbal medicines.

- Your pill planner.

- Your own medical history.

Personal pill profile

Your pill profile is a list of all the medications that you are taking—prescription drugs, over-the-counter medications, herbs, vitamins, and supplements—along with how much you are taking, how many pills you should take a day and at what

times, when you should stop taking it, and possible side effects. If you take more than two or three pills a day, you should have a pill profile to give to each doctor that you see, as well as to any family or friends who might need to be involved in your health care.

If something were to happen to you, this information would give anyone treating you a big head start.

Make several copies of the chart below to create your own personal pill profile.

Patient's name

Drug name and strength	Purpose	Pill shape/color
Dosage	Date to stop	
Dangerous side effects to report	Special instructions (take with food, missed doses, etc.)	

Drug name and strength	Purpose	Pill shape/color
Dosage	Date to stop	
Dangerous side effects to report	Special instructions (take with food, missed doses, etc.)	

Drug name and strength	Purpose	Pill shape/color
Dosage	Date to stop	
Dangerous side effects to report	Special instructions (take with food, missed doses, etc.)	

Personal pill planner

One hour before eating, not with milk, never with blood-pressure medication, three times a day, before bed, before breakfast. These instructions are meaningless until you translate them into your own lifestyle. When your doctor says, **Take with meals**, you might eat six meals a day or only two. A meal to you might be a glass of milk and a graham cracker or a seven-course smorgasbord. Not

everyone gets up at 7 am and goes to bed at 10 pm.

So, when your doctor says, **Take at bed time**, it's up to you to tell your doctor that you go to bed at 2 am.

It's no surprise that at least 50% of prescription drugs aren't taken correctly.

A pill planner can help in making sure your doctor's instructions are translated correctly.

Below is a daily schedule to record what to take and when. It should include every pill you take—prescription, over-the-counter, herbs, and vitamins—as well as when you regularly rise, eat meals, and go to bed.

Make copies of the chart below so that when your medications change, you can update your pill planner.

Patient's name

Time	Medication(s)	Special instructions (take with meals, not with grapefruit juice, etc.)
Early am		
6 am		
7 am		
8 am		
9 am		
10 am		
11 am		
12 noon		
1 pm		
2 pm		
3 pm		
4 pm		
5 pm		
6 pm		
7 pm		
8 pm		
9 pm		
10 pm		
11 pm		
12 midnight		
Late night		

Symptom list

Have you ever forgotten to tell your doctor an important symptom? The way to combat symptom amnesia is to write your symptoms down before you get to the doctor's office. Be sure to note how severe they are, when they occur, and whether or not they seem to correspond to any new medications you are taking. Then, when your doctor comes in and asks how you are doing, you've got the answer in writing.

Medical history

If you're bored filling out the same information over and over or have trouble remembering details from your distant medical past, why not write your own medical history, including your medication history, and make copies to hand out each time you visit a new doctor? The next time you visit a doctor, ask for a blank form or create your own. Also, take a copy of your pill planner, so if your doctor prescribes new medications, he/she can help place it on your schedule.

You'll have more time to read magazines or watch the goldfish in the waiting room on your next visit.

If you want to create your own medical history, be sure to include:

- Your name, address, birth date, height, and weight

- Insurance information

- Past illnesses and inherited conditions: List previous illnesses or conditions, hospitalizations, and surgeries, including head injuries, thyroid problems, seizures, heart problems, stomach problems (e.g., ulcers), diabetes, asthma. How and when were you treated and what was the result?

- Current conditions: What's bothering you? When did it start? List any details you can about the condition, such as is it worse in the morning, before eating, or after eating?

- Over-the-counter, prescription medications, vitamins, herbs, or supplements: This includes antibiotics, asthma medications, antidepressants, allergy medications, aspirin, cold medicines, estrogen, grapefruit juice (interacts with several drugs), heart medications, herbs, pain killers, and vitamins.

If you have trouble remembering details from your distant medical past, why not write your own medical history and make copies to hand out each time you visit a new doctor?

What does my doctor need to know about me?

- Smoking habits: Smoking affects the way your body uses certain medications.

- Medication history (especially drugs taken in the past associated with adverse side effects).

- Alcohol consumption, which includes beer and wine: (Combining alcohol and some drugs can be potentially fatal. Alcohol also can affect how your body responds to drugs.)

- Food, drug, or environment allergies (name allergen and describe symptoms)

- Stresses: (List any traumatic event, such as a loved one dying or retiring from a job. These events can affect not only your mental well-being but also your physical health.)

Remember, practice full disclosure. Give your doctors the information they need to treat you.

Ask Questions
Here's what you need to ask before starting on a new medication:

Risks and benefits
- Why has this medication been prescribed?

- What can I expect this medication to do for me and how does it work?

- Are there any behavioral or dietary changes I could make to treat this problem?

- What might happen if I didn't take this medicine? (This is the question that helps with the risk-benefit analysis. You may be surprised at the answers.)

- What are the short and long-term side effects?

- Which side effects signal dangerous reactions, and what should I do if they occur?

- How will this interact with other drugs I am taking?

- Can you give me any written information so I can learn more about this drug? Ask for the drug class and for the generic name. (Knowing the drug class can be helpful in case information arises about another drug in the same class that may have parallels to your own. The generic name will help in case you need to

Don't be afraid to ask

Despite the complexities of medications, far too few people ask their doctor for the information they need to take prescriptions correctly. The Massachusetts Board of Registration in Pharmacy estimates that only 4% of patients ask their doctor any questions about prescribed medications.

IT'S NO SURPRISE THAT AT LEAST **50%** OF PRESCRIPTION DRUGS AREN'T TAKEN CORRECTLY.

locate medication in an emergency or while traveling in a foreign country.)

Dosage and scheduling

- What is the dose and how many times a day should I take it?

- At what times should I take it? (Pull out your pill planner and ask the doctor to pencil in the best times.)

Safety Tip

If your weight changes by more than 10% up or down, you should always have your medications re-evaluated.

Doctors often base your dose on your weight.

- Should I take with food or without? Are there any foods or beverages, like grapefruit juice, that may interact with this? What about alcohol?

- Are there activities to avoid?

- If I were to travel, would this affect how I take this medicine?

- What should I do if I forget a dose? (It's important to ask because the answer will change depending on the drugs you take. A dose should be skipped in some cases and taken as soon as you remember in others.)

- When can I expect to see results? How long should I wait to report if it's not working?

- When should I stop taking the medication or when should I have my progress reviewed?

- Can I get a refill and how often?

- How should I store this drug?

Remember to practice full disclosure. Give your doctors the information they need to treat you.

Cost issues

- Are there any less expensive medications for my condition? It's better to bring price up with your doctor than not fill a prescription at the pharmacy because it costs too much.

- Does this drug come in generic form and is the generic acceptable?

- Are there other ways I can save money on this?

Do Not Accept Illegible Prescriptions

If you can't read it, don't expect the pharmacist to either. Always ask your doctor to print or type out the prescription. Poor penmanship may be a frequent occurrence among busy physicians, but it is an inexcusable cause of adverse consequences for patients. Also, ask your doctor to put the purpose for the drug on the label, along with information on proper use. This is especially important for those on multiple drugs. It also makes it easier for friends and family if they are involved in your care.

Find a Good Pharmacist
Choose your pharmacists as carefully as you choose your doctor. Pharmacists are a rich source of information and a last critical safety checkpoint between you and your pills. You can use pharmacists to minimize errors in much the same way hospitals do.

Get a Drug Evaluation
Anyone who is taking multiple medications could benefit from a complete drug evaluation, which is best done by a clinical pharmacist as opposed to a dispensing pharmacist. This is like a complete physical only it's done with your pills instead of your person. It involves a thorough assessment of all the prescription drugs, over-the-counter medications, herbs, dietary supplements, vitamins, and minerals that you take. Clinical pharmacists can be recommended by your doctor, the nearest teaching hospital, or the American Society of Consultant Pharmacists in Alexandria, VA, at **703.739.1300** or online at **www.ascp.com**.

If you can't afford a private consultation with clinical pharmacist, there are other means of having your medications assessed. There are several online sources for medication assessments, and some healthcare web sites have pill checkers that will point out negative interactions.

Whether you get a private drug evaluation, go online, or depend on your pharmacy to uncover problems, make sure that your medications are evaluated on a regular basis.

Buying Drugs

Buy All Your Drugs at the Same Pharmacy
This will help ensure that you aren't put on conflicting medications by oversight. Most

What do I need to know before I begin taking a new medication?

Case Study

Dorothy is a well-informed, 73-year-old woman and a careful patient. She always asks, "What happens if I don't...?" when her doctor suggests taking a new pill.

Sometimes, she decides the risks aren't worth it. Recently, her doctor prescribed an antihistamine and Prednisone (a cortisone drug) to treat a bad case of poison ivy on her arms and legs. Dorothy was wary of taking cortisone, so she started asking questions. The doctor told her that not taking the Prednisone wouldn't jeopardize her health, but that the rash would probably last longer. He also said the antihistamine would reduce the itching. At this point, Dorothy was able to do her own risk/benefit analysis.

The risk of taking the Prednisone was not worth the benefit of speeding up the healing to Dorothy, so, with her doctor's okay, she left with only the antihistamine, which would help her tolerate the rash a little longer. The rash completely disappeared after three weeks.

When her doctor tells her that not treating a minor infection could lead to a more serious infection, Dorothy conscientiously takes prescribed antibiotics. She believes in medicine, but she also believes in taking as little of it as is absolutely necessary—a hallmark of an informed patient.

pharmacies have software programs that will
check for interactions.

Ask to See the Pharmacist

You've got another opportunity to double-check
information or ask the questions your doctor
didn't answer. Take the bottle out of the package
and ask him or her to verify that this is the cor-
rect medication. Does the dosage seem to be
right? What are the side effects? Are there any
special instructions for taking the medication?
What drugs, foods, herbs, vitamins, or beverages
might affect or interact with this medicine? Does
this drug interact with any other prescriptions,
over-the-counter medications, herbs, vitamins,
food, or drink?

Request a Patient Insert

Some drug manufacturers distribute written
information to consumers in the form of
patient inserts. The **FDA** has a goal that at least
75% of people receive these inserts with new
prescriptions. By year 2006, the goal is 95%.

Pay Attention

Color, shape, and size are also clues as to whether
you have the right medication.

For purposes of safety and to distinguish
their products in the marketplace, all pharmaceutical companies want to make their pills look
different from their competitors. If you've ever
wondered why pills look the way they do, their
appearance is usually based on input from the
research and development, marketing, and regu-
latory divisions in pharmaceutical companies.

Paul Skultety, executive director of pharma-
ceutics at **Quintiles**, which does research and
development for pharmaceutical companies,
explains here how pills come to look the way
they do.

Color

The color of a drug is often chosen to distinguish
the medication from others in the same category.
Skultety was involved in developing Allegra, an
allergy medicine sold by **Hoescht Marion
Roussell**. Its competitors were Claritin and
Zyrtec, which are both small white tablets, so
Allegra became a two-tone pink capsule.

Shape

The shape of a drug can be influenced by marketing and/or manufacturing. In theory, elongated or elliptical shaped pills are easier to swallow than round ones. Unusual shapes can enhance brand recognition. Zantac is shaped like a pentagon. Inderal is shaped like a hexagon. Visken is heart-shaped. Zocor looks like a police badge.

Size

At **Quintiles**, size depends on the ingredients. **We try to formulate the smallest size possible,** says **Skultety**. **Allegra is a large capsule because of its properties. Sometimes, ingredients aren't compressible or aren't widely bioavailable.** That means **usable,** so the pills must contain a larger quantity of the compound.

Tablet versus capsule

The choice is usually company preference or tradition. Sometimes, the bitter taste of an ingredient can be masked in a capsule. **Capsules can also be the fastest way to get a pill to market**, says **Skultety**. Film coated tablets and capsules are equal from a cost standpoint, while uncoated tablets are the cheapest.

Saving Money

Prescription drug expenditures were expected to reach nearly $120 billion in the U.S. in the year 2000, second only to physician services in the nation's healthcare budget. Insurers and HMOs now pay more for prescription drugs than for hospitalizations, according to an article in **The New York Times** (11/14/99). The high tab has fueled big increases in spending for over-the-counter medicines, as well, which jumped from $10 billion in 1987 to $20 billion in 1996.

    Randall J. Wright, a pharmacist in Kansas City who lectures frequently on what consumers can do to take medicines more safely and smartly, offers these tips on how to save money on medications:

- Always ask your doctors about the cost of a medication (although they often don't know), and, if this is an issue, request the lowest cost drug available.

- Ask your doctor for drug samples. Pharmaceutical companies blanket physicians with

Pharmacists are not foolproof

According to a **U.S. News & World Report** investigation in 1996, more than half of 245 pharmacies failed to warn consumers against the dangers of mixing prescription drugs, after consumers were sent into the pharmacies with three prescriptions known to cause adverse reactions. About one third of pharmacists did not alert consumers to the potentially severe and widely publicized interaction between Hismanal, a common antihistamine, and Nizoral, an often-prescribed antifungal drug, which can cause irregular heartbeat, cardiac arrest, and sudden death.

samples. This is especially convenient for trying out a new prescription.

- Ask for a generic equivalent if you are living in a state where this is permitted.

- Where possible, ask if there is an over-the-counter substitute.

- When you get a new prescription, ask for just a few pills to try it out instead of a whole bottle. That way you won't be stuck if the medication doesn't work out. (Don't try this if you have prescription drug coverage with a co-pay.)

- Ask for a senior citizen discount.

- Buy pills in larger quantities for ongoing conditions after you know that you can tolerate the medication well, but make sure you get only enough to use before the expiration date.

- Always compare prices, whether you buy drugs in a drugstore, online, or via mail order. Prices of prescription drugs have been known to vary by as much as 91% from pharmacy to pharmacy, while prices of over-the-counter medications can vary by as much as 175%. If you find a drug cheaper elsewhere, ask your regular pharmacist if he or she can match the price.

- Phone ahead. By calling first for prices, you identify yourself as a concerned price shopper. It may get you a better deal than if you went into the store to ask—and saves on gas as well.

Safety Tip

When buying drugs online, look for the **VIPPS**. The **National Association of Boards of Pharmacy** has a certification program for online pharmacies called **Verified Internet Pharmacy Practice Sites (VIPPS)**. It requires that pharmacies be licensed in every state they ship drugs, meet patient privacy, security, and quality assurance standards, and have communication between patients and pharmacists. VIPPS-certified web sites include **drugstore.com,** Merck-Medco RX Services (**www.merck-medco.com**), **planetrx.com, and cvs.com.**

You can also contact the National Association of Boards of Pharmacy (**www.nabp.net**) to see if a site has a valid pharmacy license. For information, call **847.698.6227.**

- Click around. A study conducted at the **University of Pennsylvania Medical School** found that online prices for prescription drugs aren't always in line with market standards. The median price of Viagra by Internet was

$5.49 per pill, with prices ranging from $4.50 to $28.40. In Philadelphia drugstores, the median price was $4.50 per pill, with a range from $4.30 to $6.45.

- Consider using a mail-order service.

- When buying over-the-counter medications, ask the pharmacist if the store brand or discount brand is acceptable.

- Ask if you can get a discount for paying by cash instead of credit card.

- Call your local chapter of the **American Association for Retired Persons (AARP)** and your local disease-related organizations (for diabetes, arthritis, etc.). They may have drugs available at discount prices.

- Some pills—NEVER gelcaps or capsules— can be cut in half. Sometimes a double-strength dose costs much less than twice as much as the lower dose. So ask your doctor if this is possible with your medication. Then you need to buy a pill cutter to cut the pills in half. Warning: This only works with certain medications, such as Cardizem, Tenormin, Zantac, and Zoloft.

- Ask what you can do to help the medicine work better. Sometimes improving your diet or getting more exercise will make a difference.

Generics Versus Brands

A patent on a drug lasts 17 years from the date of filing. Once it has expired, other companies may seek **FDA** approval to offer a competitive equivalent under their own brand name. The differences among these brand-name medications are often negligible, although manufacturers often try to distinguish their product by giving it a memorable name, packaging it in a particularly appealing way, or offering it in a convenient or easy-to-digest form. However, switching between brands may be ill-advised in particular cases, so be sure to ask your pharmacists to explain differences, if they exist.

Generic medications tend to be less expensive than their brand-name equivalents— anywhere from 25 to 80 percent less. The price

Unless you have an allergy to a particular dye, the generic should be just as effective as the brand medication.

gap does not reflect a difference in quality as much as a difference in marketing and advertising costs. The **FDA** requires that generics have the same active ingredients, recommended dosages, absorption properties, and effects as the brand-name version. Variations are allowed in inactive ingredients, such as colorants or fillers. So, unless you have an allergy to a particular dye, the generic should be just as effective as the brand in most cases. Some people just can't resist the designer label and think that if they are paying more for a brand-name medication it must be better. This is more the influence of branding than reality. Most pharmacists will dispense the generic version of a drug unless your doctor specifies that you should be given a particular brand-name product by noting on the prescription to **dispense as written**. However, laws regarding the pharmacist's ability to substitute generics or other brand-name versions vary from state to state.

Do you take too many laxatives?

How often do you have a bowel movement? Once a day? Three times a day? Three times a week? If you answered "yes" to any of these choices, you are normal. Surprised? A lot of people, especially older adults, are. Many people believe that being "regular" means having one bowel movement every day. Unfortunately, this misperception often leads to the overuse of over-the-counter laxatives.

Constipation also leads many people to believe prematurely that they need a laxative. Elderly patients are prone to dehydration, which can lead to constipation. In many cases, the constipation can be treated by making a few simple changes to one's daily routine.

- Drink six to eight glasses of water a day.
- Add more fiber to your diet: eat more fresh fruits and vegetables, bran cereal, and other high-fiber foods.
- Exercise regularly.

Of course, some people really do need laxatives. If you're constipated and have been unable to find relief through these simple recommendations, the occasional use of a laxative may be necessary. Laxatives come in a variety of different forms, all of which clean out the bowel.

- Bulk-forming laxatives (such as Metamucil) increase the volume and water content of stools, making them softer and easier to pass. They typically work in 12 to 72 hours.
- Stool softeners (such as Colace) increase the wetness of the stool to make it softer and easier to pass. Oral forms work in 12 to 72 hours.
- Lubricants (such as mineral oil) oil the contents of the intestinal tract, softening the stool and making it easier to pass. Oral forms usually work in six to eight hours.
- Stimulants (such as Dulco-lax) cause rhythmic contractions of the small or large intestine to trigger bowel movements. Oral forms work in six to 12 hours.

- Saline laxatives (such as Fleet enemas) increase water in the intestines and work in 30 minutes to six hours.
- Hyperosmotic laxatives (such as Doxidan) attract water into the stool and usually work within one hour.

Older individuals should use saline laxatives or other enema products with caution. These drugs sometimes can cause other problems, such as heart failure or high blood pressure.

Laxatives are not meant for long-term use. Signs that you have misused a laxative include dehydration, abdominal cramping, constipation, diarrhea, nausea, vomiting, and bloating. See your doctor if you need to use laxatives regularly to have a bowel movement.

Taking and Storing Medications

Taking Your Medications

The first step is remembering to take your medicine. Here are some tips:

Keep your pill planner close by and look at it often.
Leave notes on your bathroom mirror or refrigerator.

Set the alarm on your watch or use a medication reminder.
Consumers can buy watch- or beeper-like alarms that can be programmed to sound each time a pill should be taken. A good selection is available through www.epill.com or 800.549.0095.

Get a container with sections for days of the week.
Use an egg carton with each cup numbered with an hour of the day. Then each morning put the pills in the cup at the time you are supposed to take them. This method won't work for certain medications that shouldn't be exposed to open air or in households where there are children who might get into the container.

Subscribe to a pill-reminder service.
For about $20 a month, you can employ a service to call you when it's time to take your medicine. One free service is available online. Go to www.mrwakeup.com and click on **Dr. Dose**.

Hard to Swallow?

Here are two methods for making pills go down easier from 50+: the Graedons' People's Pharmacy for Older Adults.

Method 1
If your pills float, instead of tipping your head back—which will cause the pill to float to the front of your mouth—try tipping it forward. This will cause the pill to go to the back of your throat where it's easier to swallow. Tricky at first, but it works.

Method 2
Put your pill in your mouth and take a drink from a bottle of soda. Keep contact with the bottle and your lips with a sucking motion. This action activates the reflex swallowing motion. Good-bye pill. You won't even know it's gone.

Traveling with Drugs

If you can't arrange to leave your illness at home when you travel, here are some suggestions that will make it easier for you to take your pills on the road:

Pack the pills first.

That way you won't forget. Buying a toothbrush in a strange place is a lot easier than buying prescription medication. Also, always keep pills in their original containers.

Carry extra pills.

Bring enough for the entire trip plus an extra two or three days—in case you are delayed.

Keep them with you.

If traveling by air, keep your medicines in your carry-on luggage. Recovering lost checked baggage can take several days.

Be prepared.

Bring a copy of all your prescriptions for emergency refills. Make sure to write down both the generic and trade name.

If you're taking large quantities of medication (for an extended trip), get a letter from your doctor explaining why you are taking the drugs. This may allay the suspicions of customs' officials.

Safe Drug Storage

The way you maintain and store your medications can be as important as how you take them. Here's what you should keep in mind:

Medicine doesn't last forever.

Over-the-counter medications usually have expiration dates, but prescription drugs commonly don't. Ask your pharmacist to write the expiration date directly on the bottle. A good rule of thumb to follow is to keep drugs for no

> Over-the-counter medications usually have expiration dates, but prescription drugs commonly don't. A good rule of thumb to follow is to keep drugs for no more than one year.

Safety Tip

If you are carrying around a lot of pills in your bag, make sure you don't leave it near curious children. You don't want your kids or grandkids to overdose on your heart medications.

more than one year. Pills can become weaker over time or break down into harmful by-products. While most medicines become less effective over time, some get more powerful. Alcohol-based cough medicine, for example, gets more potent as the liquid evaporates. A few, such as tetracyline antibiotics, are dangerous after the expiration date.

When in doubt, throw them out.
Regardless of the expiration date, if pills or liquids smell foul or change color, throw them out. Other signs that your medicines are past their prime are cracked coatings or powdered rings in bottles containing liquid medications.

The medicine cabinet is usually the worst place to keep medication.
Heat and humidity hasten chemical breakdown, and light can also affect drugs, so it's better to keep medicines in a dark and dry place, like a closet. Unless specifically directed, it's best not to store drugs in the refrigerator, either. Some medicines, such as insulin, should never be frozen.

Never keep medicines in your car.
It gets too hot in the summer and too cold in the winter.

Side Effects
You can do a great deal to minimize your chance of experiencing a side effect.

The first step is to play a more informed, active role when it comes to your pills. After all, no one cares as much as you do about the medicines you take.

Patients need to have honest discussions with their physicians about whether a drug is appropriate, says **Mike Hatch**, a clinical pharmacist with **UnitedHealthcare**. The expectation that you need a drug for every ache and pain is not realistic. You have to weigh benefits against risks. If you have a runny nose and take a decongestant, it may dry up your nose, but it can also raise your blood pressure and heart rate.

Playing a More Active Role Doesn't Mean Practicing Medicine

It means:

- Knowing what medicines you take, why you take them, how to take them correctly, and when to stop taking them.

- Working with your doctors and pharmacists to minimize your risks of drug reactions.

- Staying informed about interactions between drugs, food, alcohol, and dietary supplements.

- Taking your medications as directed.

Prescription Drugs

The side effects, drug interactions, and warnings listed for most prescription drugs are longer than a Dickens novel and scarier than a Stephen King film.

Warnings tend to provoke two responses. One, you ignore them all and pop the pill, figuring your doctor wouldn't tell you to take something that could harm you. Two, you swear off medicines altogether.

Neither of these leads to the best health outcomes.

The best response is to make sure you understand both the benefits and the risks of your medications, so that you can make informed decisions about your care as a partner with your health professionals.

Over-the-Counter Medications and Herbs

Let's face it. We're not all doctors. So it's not surprising that many of us have, at least once in our lives, misdiagnosed an illness and taken the wrong over-the-counter medication. And since most of us don't consult a doctor when buying an over-the-counter drug, mistakes can happen. Some mistakes are harmless, others can be life-threatening.

A study conducted by the Nonprescription Drug Manufacturers Association found that 12 self-treatable conditions are responsible for about 60% of over-the-counter drug sales in the U.S.: allergy, headache, arthritis, rash, sinusitis,

Synthroid
Floxin

What's in a name?

All drugs have a generic name, which is designated during its development by an organization called the **US Adopted Name Council**. This council consists of representatives from the **American Medical Association**, the **American Pharmaceutical Association**, and the **US Pharmacopoeia**.

Pharmaceutical companies choose the registered trade name, or brand name, for marketing purposes, trying to pick one that's easy to remember, like Synthroid for levothyroxine sodium or Floxin for ofloxacin. Drugs also have chemical names, which you're lucky you don't have to remember.

common cold, athlete's foot, jock itch, heartburn/indigestion, backache, acne, and vaginal yeast infection.

Here are some tips reducing the risk of taking the wrong OTC medication:

Ask Your Pharmacist
Pharmacists know more than anyone about prescription and over-the-counter drugs.

Do Your Own Research
Research alternatives to drug therapy for your health problem. For example, many digestive disorders can be relieved by reducing stress, maintaining a well-balanced, healthful diet, cutting down on caffeine and alcohol, and exercising regularly.

Pay Attention
Read the drug label carefully and thoroughly. Look for name brands and make sure there is an address and phone number on the bottle to contact if there are problems.

Consult Your Physician or Primary-Care Health Professional
If you are experiencing a condition for the first time and have just guessed what it might be, consult your physician before treating yourself with an over-the-counter drug or herbal preparation.

Medicine Is Medicine: Herbs and Supplements
Whenever you think about what drugs you take, you should always remember to include herbs, vitamins, and dietary supplements. In the minds of many, there is the impression that there are two kinds of drugs—conventional medicine and alternative or natural substances—and that neither have anything to do with the other. Nothing could be farther from the truth.

Arsenic is natural
Just because a drug is natural doesn't mean it's harmless. Arsenic, strychnine, and hemlock are all 100% natural, and small amounts of them can kill you.

There is no question that many natural substances can be medicinally effective. More than

There is no question that many natural substances can be medicinally effective. More than 25% of conventional medicines listed in the Physicians' Desk Reference are derived from natural substances.

25% of conventional medicines listed in the **Physicians' Desk Reference** are derived from natural substances. The cancer drug Taxol comes from yew tree bark; the heart drug digitalis from the foxglove plant; and aspirin from willow bark

Safety Tip

Treat herbs and supplements just like drugs and keep informed about side effects and interactions they may have with other medications. That means don't let store clerks prescribe your medicine and always report every single vitamin, herb, and supplement you take to your doctor, along with other prescription medications and over-the-counter drugs. Be sure to report everything to your anesthesiologist if you are going to have surgery. This can prevent potentially life-threatening interactions.

Just because a drug is natural doesn't mean it's harmless. Arsenic, strychnine, and hemlock are all 100% natural, and small amounts of them can kill you.

(although now it's made synthetically). Premarin, one of the most prescribed drugs in America, comes from pregnant horse (mare) urine, thus the name **pre-mar-in**.

Most herbs, supplements, and other natural remedies, however, have yet to be carefully examined in humans to assess safety and efficacy.

Herbs and supplements to avoid:

Chaparral. Suspected of causing liver damage, this herb is used for a variety of conditions from arthritis to sexually transmitted diseases.

Comfrey root. Used to purify blood and treat ulcers, but evidence suggests it can cause liver cancer.

Ephedra. Also called ma huang or epitonin, this herb contains stimulants that can raise blood pressure, cause palpitations, nerve damage, stroke, and memory loss. It can also dangerously boost the effects of stimulants in asthma drugs and decongestants. Several states limit its sale.

Germander. This weight-loss remedy has been implicated in hepatitis outbreaks.

Lobelia. In low doses, this herb (also called Indian tobacco) dilates bronchi in the lungs and enhances breathing. Larger amounts could reduce breathing, lower blood pressure, cause rapid heartbeat, coma, or death.

Pokeroot. This highly toxic herb is used for arthritis, cancer, swollen breasts, and has caused severe illness.

Sassafras. Studies have shown this herb—touted as a blood purifier and anti-infective—caused cancer in rats and mice. Once used to flavor a beverage by the same name, it's now banned.

Yohimbe. Sold as a men's aphrodisiac, this herb, which is also sold as a prescription drug (Yohimbine), can cause weakness, fatigue, stomach disorders, paralysis, and death. Some states have banned selling this without a prescription.

Special Effects: Drugs and the Older Adult

Older adults experience such a disproportionately high rate of negative drug reactions for several reasons:

Drugs stay in the body longer

Older bodies, with older livers and kidneys, are less efficient at processing and excreting drugs, so the drugs remain in the body for longer periods, increasing the risk of side effects.

More drugs mean more reactions

Older adults are much more likely to be polypharmaceutical, which means taking multiple medications, which increases the odds of bad reactions. According to figures from **AARP**, adults 65 and over represent 13% of the U.S. population, but purchase over 33% of all prescription medications. Americans over the age of 50 purchase 66% of all prescription drugs. The **Merck Manual of Geriatrics** estimates the average older adult takes seven medications a day (including over-the-counter). If you are taking five medicines a day, you have a 50% chance of having a serious drug reaction.

Lack of information on effects of drugs on older adults

Historically, older adults have been underrepresented or omitted altogether from drug testing, so age-related reactions aren't discovered until after drugs are on the market. It wasn't until 1997 that the **FDA** required drug companies to have a **Geriatric Use** section in their labeling with information about how the drugs work on elderly people.

ACCORDING TO FIGURES FROM AARP, ADULTS **65 and over** REPRESENT **13%** OF THE U.S. POPULATION, BUT PURCHASE OVER **33%** OF ALL PRESCRIPTION MEDICATIONS. AMERICANS **over the age of 50** PURCHASE **66%** OF ALL PRESCRIPTION DRUGS.

One dose for all hurts older adults

The one-dose-for-all method used today to dispense drugs is often to blame for why the same drug makes one person well and another sick. According to **Goth's Medical Pharmacology, many adverse reactions probably arise from failure to tailor the dosage of drugs to widely different individual needs.** Poly-pharmaceutical older adults are the ones most likely to suffer. New research suggests that many drugs might be effective at lower than the recommended dose.

Drug reactions mimic diseases

As a consequence of age, older adults commonly experience symptoms such as unsteadiness, heart problems, incontinence, and constipation. So what may actually be a drug reaction could easily get passed off as a condition associated with aging that might prompt a doctor to prescribe more medication. Many drugs can cause symptoms of depression. Yet rather than take people off the pill causing the symptoms, doctors may add an antidepressant to the mix. This can quickly lead to over-medication.

The Short Course In Spotting Side Effects

As a pill-taker, you are in the best position to spot potential adverse drug reactions at their earliest and least harmful stages. After all, you're going to feel side effects first and what you do about them will, in a large part, influence your health.

The most dangerous problems usually occur when two substances interact. Negative interactions can be produced by drug/drug, drug/food, drug/drink combinations. It doesn't matter whether the substances in question are prescription, over-the-counter, or dietary supplements. What counts are the chemical properties of the substances.

Here are the three main types of negative interactions that can occur:

Butting heads

The substances work against each other and cancel out the benefits—like caffeine and sleeping pills. This is called an **antagonistic** reaction.

IF YOU ARE TAKING

five MEDICINES A DAY,

YOU HAVE A

50% chance

OF HAVING A SERIOUS

DRUG REACTION.

The expectation that you need a drug for every ache and pain is not realistic. You have to weigh benefits against risks.

One, two knock-out punch

The substances work together to multiply the effects—Coumadin and aspirin are both blood thinners that when combined can result in hemorrhaging. This is called an **additive** reaction.

Surprise hit

The drugs combine to form some new reaction. Mevacor and Lopid, two cholesterol-lowering drugs, when taken together have produced on occasion a life-threatening disorder that results in muscle-tissue breakdown. This is called the 1+1=3 reaction.

And you don't need a prescription for these kinds of reactions. All three can occur from any combination of prescription drugs, over-the-counter medications, and dietary supplements.

How to recognize a reaction

Just what constitutes a negative reaction is highly subjective and hard to document. That's why it's so important that you are informed about the medications you take, what side effects have been reported in the past, and how they might interact with other substances you consume.

When you experience troubling symptoms, determining the cause requires some detective skills. Symptoms can be caused by: your medication, interaction between medications, a worsening of your condition, or by an entirely new condition.

How to Judge a Reaction

What do the symptoms mean to you? General information about physical symptoms will help you distinguish nuisance side effects from dangerous reactions, when to worry about weight loss, and the difference between normal absent-mindedness and memory loss.

What is your baseline?

That's whatever your condition was before you started the medication. Normal has to be relative to the state you are in before you take the pill. This becomes the basis for comparison and the easiest way to distinguish side effects from symptoms. If you normally have only three bowel

> Formerly when religion was strong and science weak, men mistook magic for medicine; now, when science is strong and religion weak, men mistake medicine for magic.
>
> THOMAS SZASZ
> *Psychiatrist and writer, in* The Second Sin

movements a week (your baseline), then the medication is suspect if you drop to only one or two a week. If you are mentally alert one day and think you are a zombie after taking an allergy pill, that's a pretty good indication that your problem isn't narcolepsy, it's antihistamines.

What side effects can you expect from the medication?

Make sure you understand the known side effects of the pill you are taking and when they are likely to show up. Reactions to antibiotics, for example, tend to show up quickly, sometimes only a few hours after taking the first pill. On the other hand, non-steroidal anti-inflammatories or beta blockers for high blood pressure can have subtle effects, such as memory loss, that might not show up for months.

How to Report a Reaction

Knowing the language of side effects will also help in communicating with your doctors and make it easier for them to help you.

Severity

How severe is it? That's the first question a doctor is likely to ask when you report a symptom that might be a side effect. A good rule of thumb is how much does it interfere with your ability to function? If you can go to work and do your job, if you can still play bridge without trumping your partner's trick, then your symptoms probably aren't severe. Severe is having to lie down, not being able to read or watch TV, or carry on a conversation—once again, this assumes that you could do all these things before you took the pill.

Persistence

How long has it lasted? This is the second question. A good rule of thumb for physical symptoms, such as pain or dizziness, is if it lasts more than a day or is getting progressively worse.

Common Side Effects

There are almost as many side effects as there are pills. Many—like itching, hives, rashes, sweating, vomiting—are pretty easy to recognize. Others are easy to confuse with other diseases or even life conditions. Here are some that are commonly misinterpreted along with some guidelines that will help you determine when

Make sure you understand the known side effects of the pill you are taking and when they are likely to show up.

they might signal a side effect of your medications and should be brought to your doctor's attention.

Angina

This is a lack of blood flow to heart that causes chest pain. Not all chest pain is angina, which tends to feel like a crushing, squeezing, or gripping pain in the center of the chest. It may be associated with sweating, nausea or shortness of breath. A stab or lightening bolt of pain accompanied by breathing problems might be a broken

Safety Tip

Side effects you should never ignore:
- Diarrhea or vomiting
- Breathing difficulties
- Appetite loss
- Muscle weakness
- Skin rashes
- Drowsiness or confusion
- Memory loss
- Depression
- Seizures

rib or an inflammation of the heart or lung sac. Any of these kinds of pain should be reported to your doctor immediately.

Anorexia

This is an aversion to food that can result in weight loss. It is often cited as a side effect of antidepressants, such as Prozac. Skipping lunch or losing a couple of pounds isn't a significant sign of anorexia. You should be concerned if you lose more than 5 to 10% of your body weight.

Confusion

A catch-all term, confusion shows up as a side effect of many drugs and is one of the most over-looked, because, when you are confused, you're least likely to recognize it as a side effect. Besides, who isn't confused? Life is confusion. Drug-induced confusion can show up as memory problems, inability to perform a mental task that you could before the medication (like balance a checkbook), or problems with spatial orientation. One test for confusion is to try to draw a clock face. If you have trouble placing the numbers, that's spatial confusion. Drugs can also cause problems in perceiving reality or engaging in abstract thinking. A general rule is confusion should trigger alarms when it becomes significant enough to affect daily functioning. If you go

There are almost as many side effects as there are pills.

to the store and can't remember what you wanted to buy, that's normal life confusion. If you can't remember what you do at a store or where you live, that's problematic.

Depression
While everyone knows what depression is, this can be tricky to diagnose, especially in older adults, who having lived for a longer period of time, are more likely to have experienced life events that cause sadness, the cardinal symptom of depression. Generally, depression should be considered a treatable symptom only when you experience sadness not related to a specific event or you feel worthless or suicidal.

Dizziness or vertigo
This is often confused with light-headedness. Dizziness, or vertigo, is the sensation of twirling or feeling like the room is spinning around you, while light-headedness is feeling like you will pass out (See light-headedness). Vertigo implies inner-ear or brain-stem problems and can be caused by antibiotics or drugs that affect the central nervous system.

Fatigue
This is the sensation of tiredness—but to a degree that you can still complete tasks.

Safety Tip
The action of identifying symptoms daily will make people more aware of their bodies and more adept at recognizing when a drug is making them sick and thus become more likely to stop the medication before hospitalization—or death.

Headache
If a headache is new or unusual for you and is so severe that you can't read or find relief from taking Tylenol or aspirin, you should call your doctor.

Heartburn
This usually appears as a burning in the stomach or lower chest, along with an acid-like taste in your mouth—and is almost always associated with eating or reclining.

Lethargy
Signs of this more advanced state of fatigue are having difficulty waking up or falling asleep in the middle of a conversation—when you are the one talking.

Light-headedness
If you're working in your garden, stand up suddenly and feel like you might faint or fall over, that's light-headedness. It results from insufficient blood flow or oxygen to your brain, which can be caused by many medications such as certain blood-pressure medications or treatments for congestive heart failure.

Liver failure
Early signs of liver failure include prolonged loss of appetite and dark-colored urine. Advanced symptoms are bleeding disorders and diminished mental ability.

Muscle weakness
Many heart medications can deplete potassium and magnesium. Muscle weakness is the primary sign.

Nervousness
Medications can cause restlessness, anxiety, and even panic attacks. If you suddenly experience rapid breathing, sweating, difficulties in concentrating or sitting still, tingling in your hands, or jump whenever someone enters the room—these should also be considered side effects if they represent new behavior for you.

Seizures
Typically, this is a symptom that must be recognized by someone else. In a full-blown seizure, you wouldn't necessarily know what was happening. Signs include staring and uncontrollable movements. Some people report feeling a tingling, electrical charge before the seizure begins.

Speech changes
There are four different types of speech changes that can result from medications, particularly those that affect the central nervous system. They include difficulties in producing speech, slurring words or not being able to think of a word.

Dangerous Drug Cocktails

Sometimes it's not the drug that causes the problem, but what you combine it with—be that other prescription drugs, over-the-counter medicines, food, or beverages. Scheduling your medications in a pill planner with your doctor is your first line of defense against mixing the wrong drugs together.

A case in point...
A drug approved for the treatment of Parkinson's in 1997, Mirapex, is showing promise in treating symptoms of the disease, such as tremors and rigidity. In 1999, the **American Academy of Neurology (AAN)** released data from two 3-year studies that showed Mirapex successfully controlled symptoms in more than 50% of patients—without *levodopa* (a traditional treatment), which tends to lose effectiveness over time.

Mirapex, though, comes with a very dangerous potential side effect: it could cause patients to fall asleep spontaneously. Although rare, the side effect could be fatal if it occurs in a patient driving down the interstate, so caution is advised. This goes for patients on Requip as well. These sleep attacks can occur as long as one year after beginning the drugs.

Patients on the drug may consider several precautions. Some doctors recommend that patients new to the drugs refrain from driving until they have determined how the drugs affect them. Patients are advised to consult their doctors if they feel sedated on the drugs or have sleep attacks.

If you are already taking Mirapex, call your doctor and discuss your chances of experiencing a sleep attack.

Here are some general rules for taking any kind of medicine—prescription, over-the-counter, or herbal:

Sometimes it's not the drug that causes the problem, but what you combine it with—be that other prescription drugs, over-the-counter medicines, food, or beverages.

- Take medicine with a full glass of water.

- Don't stir medicine into your food or take capsules apart (unless your doctor tells you to do so). This may change the way the drug works.

- Don't take vitamins, minerals, or herbs at the same time you take prescription drugs—they can interact with some drugs. Wait at least two hours unless your doctor or pharmacist advises otherwise.

- Don't mix medicine into hot drinks, because the heat from the drink may destroy the effectiveness of the drug.

- Never take an herb or an over-the-counter medicine with a prescription drug that performs a similar function—unless your doctor tells you to do so. For example, if you are taking sedatives, don't take Nyquil. If you are on blood thinners, don't take garlic capsules, which have blood-thinning properties. (Garlic in your food shouldn't matter unless you regularly consume more than three or four cloves a day.)

- Never chase your pills with alcohol of any kind. That means no vanilla extract shots or cough medicines, either.

Prescription/prescription reactions

The good news about prescription/prescription reactions is there are some formal systems in place to catch them. If two different doctors were to prescribe two drugs that shouldn't be taken together, some health insurers have programs in place to flag problem and some pharmacies have computerized systems that run checks when you add a prescription. This is an important reason why all prescriptions should be filled at a single pharmacy.

The bad news is that these systems aren't universal or foolproof and prescription/prescription reactions are still common. They are also the most dangerous form of interaction.

Prescription/over-the-counter reactions

Here are some specific suggestions to avoid interaction between prescription and over-the-counter drugs:

- Avoid alcohol if you are taking antihistamines, cough/cold products with the ingredient dextromethorphan or drugs that treat sleeplessness.

- Do not use drugs that treat sleeplessness if you are taking prescription sedatives or tranquilizers.

- Check with your doctor before taking products containing aspirin if you're taking a prescription blood thinner or if you have diabetes or gout.

- Do not use cough/cold or weight-control medicines with the ingredient phenylpropanolamine (PPA) if you're being treated for high blood pressure or depression, if you have heart disease, diabetes, or thyroid disease, or if you are taking other medicines containing PPA.

- Unless directed by a doctor, do not use a nasal decongestant if you are taking a prescription drug for high blood pressure or depression, or if you have heart or thyroid disease, diabetes, or prostate problems.

Prescription or over-the-counter/herb or supplement reactions

Report any side effects to doctor if severe or persistent.

Herb	Drugs to avoid	Problems caused
Black Cohosh	Hormone supplements	In high doses, it interacts to intensify effects.
Echinacea	Cortisone, cyclosporin	Could offset effects of drugs that suppress the immune system.
Ephedra	Caffeine, decongestants with stimulants	Increases risk of high blood pressure, irregular heart beat, stroke, and heart attack.
Gingko	Aspirin, anticoagulants or blood thinners, vitamin E	Increases bleeding risk because gingko has a blood-thinning effect.
Ginseng	Kava, alcohol, and drugs that affect the central nervous systems, such as Parkinson's medications, anti-psychotics, sedatives, sleeping pills	Kava enhances effects of these substances and can cause over-sedation, extreme sluggishness, and delayed responses.
Licorice	Blood pressure medications	Licorice counteracts the effects.
Ma Huang	Blood pressure medications or cold medicines that contain ephedra	Can cause sweating and nervousness, elevated blood pressure, irregular heartbeat.
St. John's Wort	Antidepressants, especially Prozac, Paxil, and Zoloft	May cause cardiac instability, delirium, and heightened reactions to stimulants, such as caffeine.
Valerian	Alcohol, sedatives, sleeping pills	Increases sedative effect.

Prescription or over-the-counter/food or drink reactions

Most everyone would guess that the wrong combination of pills might cause trouble, but few think about what they chose to swill with a pill—a glass of water, soda, milk, or grapefruit juice. This has proven to be a fatal oversight in more than a few cases. Grapefruit juice, for example, has ingredients that can make certain drugs 700% more powerful, especially heart medications like Plendil *(felodipine)* and Procardia *(nifedipine)*.

Here are some combos you should consider avoiding, unless your physician has made you aware of over-riding factors that would warrant the risks.

Report any side effects to doctor if severe or persistent.

Drug	Food or drinks to avoid	Problems caused
Aldactone	Salt substitutes containing potassium	Dangerous elevation of potassium levels.
Accupril	Alcohol, salt substitutes containing potassium.	Alcohol may increase effect. Salt substitutes can elevate potassium.
Diuretics *(like Lanoxin or digoxin)*	Black licorice	Exacerbates potassium loss, which can lead to weakness, muscle pain, paralysis, and coma.
Calcium channel blockers *(other than amlodipine and diltiazem)*	Grapefruit and grapefruit juice	A substance in grapefruit over-rides an enzyme that regulates the amount of drug absorbed. This can make your pills up to 7 times more powerful.
Capoten	Salt substitutes	(See aldactone.)
Cipro	Milk or milk products and caffeine	Milk interferes with absorption and can render drug ineffective. Cipro enhances the stimulative effects of caffeine.
Coumadin	Broccoli, brussels sprouts, cabbage, kale, kohlrabi, spinach, and liver	These foods are all rich in vitamin K, which helps blood clot. This works against the Coumadin, which seeks to inhibit clotting.
Didronel	Milk or milk products	(See Cipro.)
Dilantin	Pudding	Researchers aren't sure why, but one study found that amount of the drug in the blood stream was cut in half when patients took Dilantin in vanilla pudding to mask the taste.
Dyazide	Salt substitutes	(See Aldactone.)
Heart medications *(such as Cardene, Lipitor, Mevacor, Norvasc, Plendil, ProcardiaXL, and Zocor)*	Grapefruit juice	Exaggerates the effect of the drugs. (See calcium channel-blockers.)
Lanoxin	Oatmeal	Bran interferes with absorption and makes drug less effective.

Prescription or over-the-counter/food or drink reactions *continued*		
Drug	Food or drinks to avoid	Problems caused
Laxatives that contain bisacodyl *(such as Carter's, Dulcolax, or Fleet)*	Milk or milk products	Milk causes the pills to dissolve in the stomach instead of the small intestine.
MAO inhibitors *(such as Nardil and Parnate)*	Foods that contain tyramine, including avocados, bananas, beef liver (stored), many cheeses (especially aged), brewer's yeast, broad beans, imported beers, caviar, Chartreuse liqueur, Chianti, chicken liver (stored), chocolate (large quantities), Drambuie, over-ripe or canned figs, pickled, salted, or smoked fish, meat concentrate or pates, fermented foods like miso or soy sauce, pepperoni, salami, summer sausage, vermouth, and yeast extracts or supplements.	Tyramine, a substance in all these foods, can cause a significant, life-threatening elevation of blood pressure.
Monopril	Salt substitutes	(See Aldactone.)
Noroxin	Milk or milk products and caffeine	(See Cipro.)
Phenobarbital, primidone	Alcohol	Causes increased drowsiness.
Tetracycline-like drugs and other antibiotics *(such as amoxicillin, penicillin, Zithromax, and nitrofurantoin*	Milk or milk products	(See Cipro.)
Theophylline *(an asthma drug in Bronkaid tablets),* **Bronkodyl, Primatene tablets, Slo-bid, and Theo-Dur**	Caffeine, hot peppers, and charbroiled foods	Caffeine boosts the effects of these drugs, which can lead to overdoses. So do hot peppers. Charbroiled foods cause the drug to be eliminated more quickly, thus reducing its effectiveness.
Tylenol *(acetaminophen)* **and other pain-killers, such as Motrin** *(ibuprofen)*	Alcohol	Increases risk of liver toxicity.
Vasotec	Salt substitutes	(See Aldactone.)

Side Effects Checklist

Health researcher **Susan Steffes** has a close relationship with her grandmother and wants to make sure she stays as healthy as possible. She suspected that her grandmother might be experiencing side effects, but didn't recognize that the symptoms were from a drug she was taking. So, she created a checklist last winter when her grandmother was about to start a new prescription.

It worked wonders—within four days we knew that her symptoms were a direct result of her new medication, says Steffes. She told me afterward that she would never have realized that what she was experiencing was because of the new prescription. She just thought she wasn't feeling well; perhaps coming down with the flu or something. She discontinued the medication after consulting with her physician.

The checklist on the next page was developed from her suggestions.

Side effects checklist

Drug name	Dose	Drug start date	Today's date

Overall, how did you feel after the first day on the medication?
Note any changes in health, mood, or behavior.

Rate the following symptoms you experienced on a scale of 1 to 10, with 10 being the most severe.
All severe symptoms should be reported to your doctor immediately.

(Symptoms shown below in orange could be life-threatening.
Call your doctor before taking another dose.)

Symptom	Day 1	Day 2	Day 3	Day 4	Day 5	Day 6	Day 7
Drowsiness							
Weakness							
Problems sleeping							
Blurred Vision							
Nausea							
Changes in appetite							
Changes in sexual function							
Dry mouth							
Constipation							
Numbness or tingling							
Seizures							
Rapid or irregular heartbeat							
Problems urinating							
Rash or hives							
Breathing problems							
Other symptoms or feelings that began after taking this medication							

Digestive System

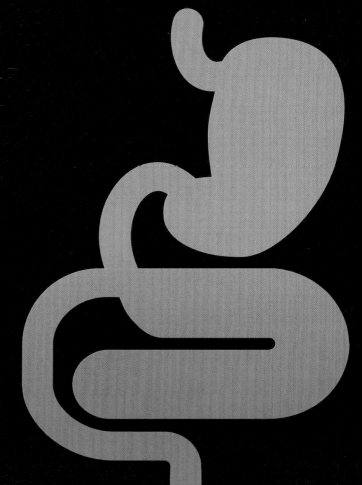

The gastrointestinal tract is home to a complex of nerves that control digestion and are, in turn, controlled by a complicated hierarchy of hormones, neurotransmitters, and connections to the brain and spinal cord.

igestion begins in the mouth, where chewing reduces food to a fine texture and an enzyme in saliva begins to convert starch into simple sugars. Swallowed food passes through the esophagus into the stomach, where hydrochloric acid kills most of the bacteria in the food. The partially processed food then passes into the small intestine. Once the nutrients from the food have been absorbed by the body, the remaining food passes into the large intestine and is turned into solid waste. It's a complicated process and full of pitfalls. Fortunately, though, new advances in research are making the digestive system easier to understand and control.

The exact mechanisms of many gastrointestinal relief agents are unknown. Some (histamine blockers and antacids) decrease stomach acid, while others (anti-inflammatories) inhibit the production of substances that produce inflammation. The anti-infectives rid the stomach of a bacterium.

In 1995, the **FDA** approved a handful of prescription heartburn relief agents for use as over-the-counter medications, making it

> **To eat is human, to digest divine.**
>
> MARK TWAIN

Digestion is a complicated process and full of pitfalls. Fortunately, though, new advances in research are making the digestive system easier to understand and control.

easier for sufferers to self-medicate as soon as symptoms appear. (However, self-medication isn't always the answer. See **The hidden danger of heartburn** on page 41 for more information.)

Many of the 21 million Americans who suffer from chronic heartburn—gastroesophageal reflux disease (GERD)—have also found symptom relief in prescription drug therapy. And antibiotics have been successful in relieving most patients of peptic ulcers. Antibiotics, for the first time, offer a cure for peptic ulcers, rather than just treating the symptoms.

Cures for many digestive disorders are not yet in hand. However, the millions of people who suffer from digestive disorders are growing increasingly comfortable as drug therapy improves.

> I would like to find a stew that will give me heartburn immediately, instead of at three o' clock in the morning.
>
> JOHN BARRYMORE

Colitis

Symptoms: diarrhea, abdominal pain, fever, fatigue, weight-loss, joint pain.

🛑 General Warnings

- **Do not combine the following drugs with alcohol.**
- **Some drugs may effectively treat ulcers, but do not preclude the possibility of stomach cancer.**

Common drugs for colitis

Report any side effects to doctor if severe or persistent. Those in orange, report immediately.

Important side effects	Negative drug interactions	Special warnings	
Asacol *(mesalamine)*, an anti-inflammatory			$$$
Dipentum *(olsalazine)*, an anti-inflammatory			$$$
Abdominal cramps, diarrhea, dizziness, increased number of loose stools, appetite loss, headache, runny nose, sneezing, rash, itching, skin or eye discoloration, back or stomach pain, chills, fast heartbeat, fever, nausea, vomiting, shortness of breath, swollen stomach, fatigue, rectal irritation	*Do not combine with:* Benemid *(probenecid)*. *Use caution with:* Azulfidine *(sulfasalazine)* and Coumadin *(warfarin)*. Consult your doctor before combining these drugs with any other drug.	*Do not use if:* you have impaired kidney function; a sulfite or aspirin allergy; active ulcer disease; or have had a varicella vaccine in the past six weeks. *Use caution if:* you are allergic to aspirin or other salicylates, olsalazine or sulfasalazine; have allergies, impaired liver function, a history of blood clotting, or low white blood cell counts. Do not chew or break tablets. Take with a meal.	

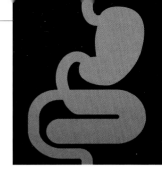

Common drugs for colitis *continued*		
Important side effects	**Negative drug interactions**	**Special warnings**
Azulfidine *(sulfasalazine)*, an anti-infective/anti-inflammatory drug **$$**		
Abdominal cramps, diarrhea, appetite loss, nausea, vomiting, aching joints and muscles, pain in back, legs or stomach, discolored fingernails, lips or skin, chest pain, cough, breathing or swallowing difficulty fever, sore throat, peeling, blistering or loose skin, bleeding, bruising, fatigue, light sensitivity	*Use caution with:* Coumadin *(warfarin)*, Dilantin *(phenytoin)*, folic acid (a B-complex vitamin), Lanoxin *(digoxin)*, and antidiabetics (Actos, Amaryl, and Avandia).	*Do not use if:* you are allergic to any sulfa drug or aspirin or have a urinary or intestinal obstruction. *Use caution if:* you have allergies, asthma, impaired liver or kidney function, a G6PD-enzyme deficiency, a history of porphyria, or a drug-induced blood cell or bone marrow disorder. Do not chew or break tablets. Take with a meal. Drink up to two quarts of water daily.
Slippery Elm		

The hidden danger of heartburn

What do you do when you have heartburn? Run to the store and pick up some Pepcid AC? That makes sense. But, what do you do when you have frequent heartburn? Run to the store and pick up more Pepcid AC? That doesn't make sense.

People who suffer from severe, frequent heartburn—also known as gastroesophageal reflux (GERD)—are at risk for developing a cancer known as esophageal adenocarcinoma. Though still rare, this type of cancer is becoming more common.

When people suffering from GERD self-medicate with any of the dozens of over-the-counter heartburn-relief agents on the market, they relieve symptoms, but they may also mask more serious diseases.

With several new and powerful over-the-counter heartburn medications on the market, it has become easier for sufferers to avoid making a trip to see their doctor. Starting in 1995, the **Food and Drug Administration** has approved the former prescription drugs Tagamet HB, Pepcid AC, Axid AR, and Zantac 75, among others, as over-the counter medications.

The best advice for anyone suffering from long-term heartburn, or who has difficulty swallowing or abdominal pain, is to see a doctor. Beyond that, here are a few tips:

- The ideal first line of defense in the prevention and treatment of heartburn is nondrug therapy, used in combination with drugs. Doctors often recommend that heartburn sufferers avoid sleeping, and even lying down, for several hours after eating; sleep with the head elevated; avoid foods that aggravate heartburn; and avoid alcohol and smoking.

- Heartburn medications don't all do the same thing. Some, such as Tagamet and Pepcid, prevent heartburn, while others, including Rolaids, Tums, and Maalox, treat acute heartburn. Ask your doctor which one is right for you.

Gastroesophageal reflux disease (GERD), heartburn, peptic ulcer

Symptoms of GERD (also called reflux): Sour taste in the mouth, especially in the morning, difficulty swallowing, belching, heartburn that gets worse after lying down.

Symptoms of heartburn: the feeling of gaseousness or fullness in the abdomen, burning sensation in the chest.

Symptoms of peptic ulcer: persistent, gnawing stomach pain relieved by eating.

🛑 General Warnings

- Do not combine the following drugs with alcohol.
- Some drugs may effectively treat ulcers, but do not preclude the possibility of stomach cancer.

Common drugs for GERD, heartburn, peptic ulcer

Report any side effects to doctor if severe or persistent. Those in orange, report immediately.

Important side effects	Negative drug interactions	Special warnings
Prevacid *(lansoprazole)*, antacid and proton pump inhibitor		$$$$
Prilosec *(omeprazole)*, antacid and proton pump inhibitor		$$$$
Diarrhea, constipation, vomiting, itching, rash, headache, dizziness, stomach pain	*Do not combine with:* alcohol. *Use caution with:* ampicillin, Antabuse *(disulfiram)*, anticoagulants *(dicumarol, Miradon, warfarin)*, Carafate *(sucralfate)*, cyclosporine, Dilantin *(phenytoin)*, iron, Lanoxin *(digoxin)*, Nizoral *(ketoconazole)*, Theo-Dur *(theophylline)*, Valium *(diazepam)*.	*Do not use if:* you have active bone marrow or blood cell disorder. *Use with caution if:* you have a history of liver disease, impaired liver function, bone marrow or blood cell disorders, or if you smoke. Take Prevacid on an empty stomach.
Alka-Seltzer *(aspirin, sodium bicarbonate)*		
Gastric swelling, gaseousness, nausea, heartburn, loss of appetite, stomach pain, black or tarry stools	*Do not combine with:* adrenocortical steroids (e.g., Azmacort, Flonase, Ultravate), alcohol, anticoagulants (e.g., Coumadin, *dicumarol*, Miradon), Depakote *(valproic acid)*, Folex *(methotrexate)*, and NSAIDs (e.g., Aleve, Daypro, Relafen). *Use caution with:* all other medications.	*Do not use if:* you have liver or kidney damage, a bleeding disorder, or a history of ulcer disease. Do not use for more than 10 days. *Use caution if:* you have congestive heart failure or high blood pressure. Contains a significant amount of sodium. Do not take without dissolving in water first.

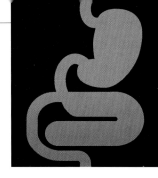

Common drugs for GERD, heartburn, peptic ulcer *continued*		
Important side effects	Negative drug interactions	Special warnings
Axid *(nizatidine)*, histamine (H2) blocker		
Pepcid *(famotidine)*, histamine (H2) blocker		
Tagamet *(cimetidine)*, histamine (H2) blocker		
Zantac *(ranitidine)*, histamine (H2) blocker		
Headache, confusion, heart changes, bleeding, bruising, fever, chills, increased infection	*Do not combine with:* alcohol. *Use caution with:* aspirin, Coumadin *(warfarin)*, Dilantin *(phenytoin)*, Halcion *(triazolam)*, and Valium *(diazepam)*.	*Use caution if:* you have impaired liver or kidney function; have a low white cell count; or a history of acute porphyria. Do not stop these drugs abruptly if they are used to treat an ulcer. After stopping, call your doctor if symptoms recur.
Pepto-Bismol *(bismuth subsalicylate)*		
Ringing in the ears	*Do not combine with:* aspirin-containing products (e.g., Bufferin). *Use caution with:* anticoagulants (e.g., Coumadin), Folex *(methotrexate)*, and Tolinase *(tolbutamide)*.	Do not use for more than two days without your doctor's consent.
Rolaids *(calcium carbonate)*		
Tums *(calcium carbonate)*		
Constipation, diarrhea, flatulence	*Do not combine with:* tetracycline, minocycline.	Do not take Rolaids for more than two weeks without your doctor's consent. Separate doses of Rolaids and other medications by at least two hours.
Licorice		
	Use caution with: adrenocortical steroids (Azmacort, Deltasone, Ultravate), *cortisol,* digitalis preparations (e.g., Cedilanid-D, Crystodigin, Lanoxin), and thiazide diuretics.	*Do not use if:* you have liver problems, congestive heart failure, poor kidney function, hypertonia, hypokalemia, or low potassium levels in your blood. Do not take licorice for more than six weeks.
Slippery Elm		

Endocrine System

The endocrine system is a network of glands that produce, store, and release various hormones to maintain our bodies' functioning. Problems arise when an endocrine gland produces too much or too little of a hormone. Because the endocrine system functions as a body regulator, it influences nearly every other part of our system. So, when something affects it, the symptoms can be many and far-ranging.

S cientists are making some newsworthy strides in their research on the endocrine system. They believe they may have found a druglike chemical that mimics the effect of insulin. For a lot of diabetics, the thought of popping an insulin pill instead of injecting the liquid form may sound too good to be true. It may not be.

Researchers are also looking into the possibility of delaying the onset of menopause. If they succeed, they could better search for the reason why menopause is often connected with osteoporosis, heart disease, and dementia.

What glands constitute the endocrine system?

Adrenal

Ovaries

Pancreas

Parathyroid

Pineal

Pituitary

Testes

Thyroid

Thymus

> I'll tell you what's wrong with my mother. She's going through mental-pause.

BROOKS BALLARD
age 10

A better understanding of the exact mechanics of menopause could lead to better treatments. For now, estrogen replacement is the primary treatment during and after menopause.

Following is a sampling of medications that treat disorders of the endocrine system.

Diabetes

Symptoms: increased thirst, hunger, urination.

 General Warnings

- These drugs are only part of a diabetes treatment program. They are not meant to replace a healthy diet and exercise.

Common drugs for diabetes

Report any side effects to doctor if severe or persistent. Those in orange, report immediately.

Important side effects	Negative drug interactions	Special warnings
Actos *(pioglitazone)*, thiazolidinediones, an antidiabetic		$$$$
Avandia *(rosiglitazone)*, thiazolidinediones, an antidiabetic		$$$$$
Dizziness, headache, nausea, vomiting, fatigue, general pain, muscle soreness, sore throat, coughing, back pain, infection, swelling of feet or legs, painful or increased urination, abdominal pain, dark urine, appetite loss, exhaustion, yellow eyes or skin, teeth problems, fever, runny or stuffy nose	*Use caution with:* adrenocortical steroids (Azmacort, Deltasone, Ultravate), alcohol, Baycol *(cerivastatin)*, calcium channel blockers (Adalat CC, Cardizem, Norvasc), cyclosporine, Halcion *(triazolam)*, Hismanal *(astemizole)*, ketoconazole, Lescol *(fluvastatin)*, Lipitor *(atorvastatin)*, Mevacor *(lovastatin)*, Neutrexin *(trimetrexate)*, Questran *(cholestyramine)*, oral contraceptives (Loestrin, Nordette, Ortho Cyclen), Pravachol *(pravastatin)*, Prograf *(tacrolimus)*, Zocor *(simvastatin)*, and all other medications.	*Use caution if:* you are over 60 years old or have unstable diabetes; or if you have an infection or a fever, a deficiency of red blood cells, liver damage, allergies, diabetic ketocidosis, Type I diabetes, heart or liver disease. A liver function test is recommended before use of these drugs. Wear an ID tag stating that you are taking this medication. This drug can cause low blood sugar, so carry a glucagon kit at all times.

Insulin in a pill?

Scientists from the United States, Spain, and Sweden are on the trail of a compound that might make it possible one day to package insulin in the form of a pill.

The researchers examined 50,000 different compounds in their search for a substance that could mimic the effects of insulin. One of the compounds they studied, L-783,281, significantly lowered the blood sugar of mice when administered by mouth. Interestingly, L-783, 281 was derived from a fungus growing on a leaf collected in the Democratic Republic of Congo.

Will Type I diabetics someday be able to swallow a pill instead of injecting themselves with insulin? It's a distinct possibility. Researchers will continue working with the compound to find ways of making it both safe and effective for human use.

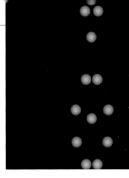

Common drugs for diabetes *continued*

Important side effects	Negative drug interactions	Special warnings

Amaryl *(glimepiride)*, an antidiabetic/sulfonylurea $

Appetite loss, dizziness, weakness, nausea, headache, sweating, restlessness, rapid pulse, anxiety, lightheadedness, poor coordination, slurred speech, confusion, sleepiness, seizures, convulsions, weakness of a part of the body, fainting

Use caution with: alcohol, aspirin and other salicylates, Benemid *(probenecid)*, beta blockers (Inderal, Sectral, Tenormin), bronchodilators (Brethaire, Proventil, Serevent), Chloromycetin *(chloramphenicol)*, corticosteroids, Dilantin *(phenytoin)*, Coumadin *(warfarin)*, diuretics, estrogen, MAO inhibitors (Marplan, Nardate, Parnate), Monistat *(miconazole)*, Nicobid *(nicotinic acid)*, Nydrazid *(isoniazid)*, nonsteroidal anti-inflammatories (Aleve, Daypro, Toradol), oral contraceptives (Loestrin, Nordette, Ortho Cyclen), phenothiazines (Compazine, Mellaril, Thorazine), sulfa drugs (Azo Gantrisin, Bactrim DS, Septra DS), and thyroid hormones (Cytomel, Synthroid).

Use caution if: you are allergic to other sulfonylurea or "sulfa" drugs; have liver or kidney disease; have experienced prolonged vomiting; cannot recognize hypoglycemia; are malnourished; have a high fever; suffer from a pituitary or adrenal insufficiency; or you have a history of congestive heart failure, peptic ulcer disease, cirrhosis of the liver, or hypothyroidism.

Glucophage *(metformin)*, an antidiabetc agent/biguanide $$$

Appetite loss, diarrhea, nausea, abdominal bloating, gas, or metallic taste, rapid and shallow breathing, sleepiness, weakness, muscle pain, abdominal distress, blurred vision, cold sweats, confusion, anxiety, rapid heartbeat, shakiness

Do not use with: alcohol.
Use caution with: adrenocortical steroids (Azmacort, Deltasone, Ultravate), alcohol, antiasthmatics (Accolate, Azmacort, Serevent), antipsychotics (Haldol, Serentil, Thorazine), calcium channel blockers (Adalat CC, Cardizem, Norvasc), Dilantin *(phenytoin)*, diuretics (Aldactone, Diamox, Lasix), *estrogen,* Lanoxin *(digoxin)*, Moduretic *(amiloride)*, *morphine, niacin,* oral contraceptives (Loestrin, Nordette, Ortho Cyclen), Procan SR *(procainamide)*, Quinidex *(quinidine)*, quinine, Rifamate *(isoniazid)*, Tagamet *(cimetidine)*, thyroid hormones (Cytomel, Synthroid), *trimethoprim,* Vancocin HCl *(vancomycin)*, and Zantac *(ranitidine)*.

Do not use if: you have impaired kidneys, liver disease, a serious infection, alcoholism, a heart or lung insufficiency, chronic metabolic acidosis or ketoacidosis, or are going to have a radiology test that uses iodinated contrast media.
Use caution if: you will have surgery soon, a kidney x-ray, or have a history of megaloblastic anemia. Glucophage may cause lactic acidosis, a build-up of lactic acid in the blood that is often fatal.

Common drugs for diabetes *continued*

Important side effects	Negative drug interactions	Special warnings

Glucotrol XL *(glipizide)*, an antidiabetic/sulfonylurea $

Important side effects	Negative drug interactions	Special warnings
Anorexia, dizziness, constipation, nausea, heartburn, changed taste in mouth, sweating, restlessness, rapid pulse, anxiety, weakness, lightheadedness, poor coordination, slurred speech, confusion, sleepiness, seizures, convulsions, weakness of a part of the body, fainting	*Use caution with:* adrenocortical steroids (Azmacort, Deltasone, Ultravate), alcohol, antacids, antiasthmatics (Azmacort, Serevent, Ventolin), antipsychotics (Haldol, Serentil, Thorazine), aspirin, Atromid-S *(clofibrate)*, Benemid *(probenecid)*, beta blockers (Inderal, Sectral, Tenormin), calcium channel blockers (Adalat CC, Cardizem, Norvasc), Chloromycetin *(chloramphenicol)*, Coumadin *(warfarin)*, Diflucan *(fluconazole)*, Dilantin *(phenytoin)*, diuretics (Diamox, Hydrodiuril, Midamor), estrogen, Lopid *(gemfibrozil)*, MAO inhibitors (Marplan, Nardil, Parnate), Monistat *(miconazole)*, Nicobid *(nicotinic acid)*, nonsteroidal anti-inflammatories (Aleve, Daypro, Toradol), Nydrazid *(isoniazid)*, oral contraceptives (Loestrin, Nordette, Ortho Cyclen), Rifadin *(rifampin)*, Sporanox *(itraconazole)*, sulfa drugs (Azo Gantrisin, Bactrim DS, Septra DS), thyroid hormones (Cytomel, Synthroid), and Tagamet *(cimetidine)*.	*Use caution if:* you are allergic to sulfonylurea or "sulfa" drugs; you have unstable diabetes; have liver or kidney impairment; don't know how to recognize hypoglycemia; or you have a history of congestive heart failure, peptic ulcer disease, cirrhosis of the liver, bone marrow depression, hypothyroidism, or porphyria.

Glyburide, an antidiabetic/sulfonylurea $$

Important side effects	Negative drug interactions	Special warnings
Anorexia, bloating, heartburn, nausea, sweating, restlessness, rapid pulse, anxiety, dizziness, weakness, lightheadedness, poor coordination, slurred speech, confusion, sleepiness, seizures, convulsions, weakness of a part of the body, fainting	*Use caution with:* adrenocortical steroids (Azmacort, Deltasone, Ultravate), alcohol, anabloic steroids, antacids, antiasthmatics (Azmacort, Serevent, Ventolin), antibiotics (Cipro, Floxin, Levaquin), anticoagulants *(dicumarol, Miradon, warfarin)*, antipsychotics (Haldol, Serentil, Thorazine), aspirin, Atromid-S *(clofibrate)*, beta blockers (Inderal, Sectral, Tenormin), calcium channel blockers (Adalat CC, Cardizem, Norvasc), Chloromycetin *(chloramphenicol)*, Diflucan *(fluconazole)*, Dilantin *(phenytoin)*, estrogen, Glucophage *(metformin)*, isoniazid,	*Use caution if:* you are allergic to sulfonylurea or "sulfa" drugs; you have unstable diabetes or G6PD deficiency; have liver or kidney problems; don't know how to recognize hypoglycemia; or have a history of problems with blood clotting, congestive heart failure, peptic ulcer disease, cirrhosis of the liver, hypothyroidism, or porphyria.

48

continued on next page

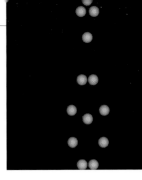

Common drugs for diabetes continued

Important side effects	Negative drug interactions	Special warnings
Glyburide continued		$
	Lasix *(furosemide)*, Lopid *(gemfibrozil)*, MAO inhibitors (Marplan, Nardil, Parnate), *niacin*, nonsteroidal anti-inflammatories (Aleve, Daypro, Toradol), Nydrazid *(isoniazid)*, oral contraceptives (Loestrin, Nordette, Ortho Cyclen), *probenecid*, Sporanox *(itra-conazole)*, sulfa drugs (Azo Gantrisin, Bactrim DS, Septra DS), Tagamet *(cimetidine)*, thiazide diuretics, and thyroid hormones (Cytomel, Synthroid).	

Menopause

Symptoms: hot flashes, night sweats, pain during intercourse, vaginal dryness, nervousness, irritability, and more frequent urination.

Common drugs for menopause

Report any side effects to doctor if severe or persistent. Those in orange, report immediately.

Important side effects	Negative drug interactions	Special warnings
Cycrin *(medroxyprogesterone)*, progestin hormones		$
Provera *(medroxyprogesterone)*, progestin hormones		$
Stomach pain, swelling of face, ankles or feet, headache, mood changes, fatigue, weight gain, abnormal menstrual bleeding, unexpected flow of breast milk, depression, rash, changes in speech, coordination or vision, shortness of breath	*Use caution with:* Cytadren *(aminoglutethimide)*, Norvir *(ritonavir)*, and Rifadin *(rifampin)*.	*Do not use if:* have liver problems, abnormal vaginal bleeding, or a history of cancer of the breast or reproductive organs. *Use caution if:* you have kidney problems, asthma, diabetes, emotional depression, epilepsy, heart disease, or migraine headaches.
Estrace Tabs *(estrogen)*, female sex hormones		$
Estraderm *(estrogen)*, female sex hormones		$$$

49

continued on next page

Common drugs for menopause *continued*

Important side effects	Negative drug interactions	Special warnings

Premarin *(estrogen)*, female sex hormones $

Prempro *(estrogen)*, female sex hormones $

Abdominal bloating, stomach cramps, appetite loss, breast changes, swelling of legs or feet, weight gain, headache, loss of coordination, vision changes, pain in chest, groin or leg, shortness of breath, slurred speech, weakness or numbness in arm or leg	*Do not use with:* tobacco *Use caution with:* adrenocortical steroids (Azmacort, Deltasone, Ultravate), anticoagulants, *(dicumarol,* Miradon, *warfarin),* anticonvulsants (Depakene, Diantin, Tegretol), antipsychotics (Haldol, Serentil, Thorazine), barbiturates (Amytal, Seconal, Solfoton), Dantrium *(dantrolene),* oral antidiabetics (Azulfidine, Gantrisin, Glucotrol), Rifadin *(rifampin),* thyroid hormones (Cytomel, Synthroid), tricyclic antidepressants (Elavil, Norpramin, Vivactil), and vitamin C.	*Do not use if:* you have liver problems, abnormal vaginal bleeding, sickle cell disease, breast cancer, estrogen-dependent cancer or a history of thrombophlebitis, embolism, heart attack, or stroke. *Use caution if:* you have had a bad reaction to estrogen therapy; have a history of breast or reproductive organ cancer or blood-clotting disorders; or have fibrocystic breast changes, fibroid tumors of the uterus, endometriosis, migraine-like headaches, epilepsy, asthma, heart disease, high blood pressure, gallbladder disease, diabetes, or porphyria; or will have surgery in the near future.

Black Cohosh

Stomach discomfort

Greater Burnet

Hormone therapy or grin and bear it?

As women begin the transition into menopause, many experience symptoms that range from annoying—increased urination, especially at nighttime—to downright painful—pain during intercourse and even urinary tract infections. The treatment options are designed to tailor-fit each individual's body.

There are three reasons for taking estrogen following the onset of menopause:

- To control the symptoms outlined above.
- To decrease the likelihood of developing osteoporosis-related bone fractures. This is the most important reason for estrogen replacement; following a hip fracture, 20% of women die within two years.

- To decrease the risk of cardiovascular disease and heart attack. The jury is still out on the connection between estrogen and cardiovascular disease. Early reports showed that women taking estrogen were at decreased risk for the disease, but head-to-head studies of estrogen versus placebo have not shown a benefit. The best advice for women entering menopause is to consult their doctors and design a treatment plan best suited to their needs.

The standard hormone therapy for the symptoms of menopause is estrogen combined with progesterone. Estrogen alone could increase the risk of endometrial cancer, but the addition of progesterone actually lowers the risk

below that of women NOT taking estrogen. Women who experience a severe loss of energy or libido may also benefit from testosterone, although evidence is scant to support this idea. Some women fear estrogen could cause breast cancer. Though the estrogen-breast cancer connection is not proven, some doctors suggest combining the hormone therapy with frequent breast exams.

One alternative option that has been receiving attention is phytoestrogen therapy. Phytoestrogens are found in soy products, including soymilk, and may ease the symptoms of menopause. Other alternative products that may relieve some symptoms include wild yams, black cohoosh root, and ginseng.

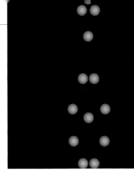

Thyroid disorders

The most common thyroid disorders are hyperthyroidism, hypothyroidism, and subacute thyroiditis.

Symptoms of hyperthyroidism (overproduction of thyroid hormone): weight loss, increased appetite, increased heart rate or blood pressure, nervousness, and sweating, frequent bowel movements, diarrhea, muscle weakness, trembling hands, and the development of a goiter.

Symptoms of hypothyroidism: lethargy, reduced heart rate, increased sensitivity to cold, tingling or numbness in hands, and the development of a goiter.

Symptoms of subacute thyroiditis: (symptoms often appear after a viral infection) pain in thyroid gland, thyroid feels tender to the touch, pain when swallowing or turning the head.

Common drugs for thyroid disorders

Report any side effects to doctor if severe or persistent. Those in orange, report immediately.

Important side effects	Negative drug interactions	Special warnings
Levoxyl *(levothyroxine)*, hypothyroid agents		$
Synthroid *(levothyroxine)*, hypothyroid agents		$
Headache, rash, hives, heartbeat changes, chest pain, shortness of breath. Signs of overdose include headache, palpitations, chest pain, heat intolerance, sweating, leg cramps, weight loss, diarrhea, vomiting, nervousness	*Use caution with:* androgens, antacids containing aluminum hydroxide, antiasthmatics (Accolate, Azmacort, Serevent), anticoagulants *(dicumarol,* Miradon, *warfarin)*, antidepressants (Elavil, Nardil, Prozac), antidiabetics *(insulin,* Glucotrol, Micronase), Carafate *(sucralfate),* Colestid *(colestipol),* diet medications, digitalis preparations (Cedilanid, Crystodigin, Lanoxin), *epinephrine* injections, iron, Questran *(cholestyramine),* and soy products.	*Do not use if:* you have an adrenal insufficiency or are using it to lose weight and your thyroid function is normal. These drugs should not be used to treat nonspecific fatigue, obesity, infertility, or slow growth. *Use caution if:* you have high blood pressure, heart disease, or diabetes or a history of Addison's disease.

Heart and Circulatory

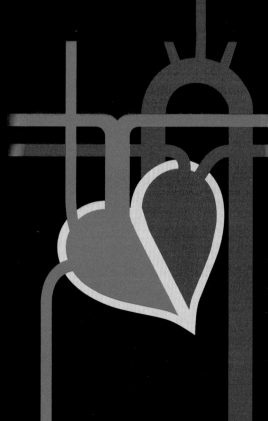

Each day the average heart "beats" (or expands and contracts) 100,000 times and pumps about 2,000 gallons of blood.

ach time the heart contracts, the left ventricle pumps blood into the aorta, which then sends the blood throughout the body. On its trip through the body, the blood drops off oxygen and picks up carbon dioxide. It then heads back to the heart, where it enters the right atrium, then streams into the lungs, where it picks up new oxygen and repeats the whole process. That's a lot of work for a small organ.

In matters of the heart, there's good news and there's bad news. Deaths due to heart attack and stroke have fallen in the US in the past several years. Early detection of heart disease is becoming easier and treatment is becoming better.

The bad news is the increasing survival rates of heart attack victims are contributing to increasing death rates from congestive heart failure, a term that refers to the reduced ability of the heart to pump enough blood to provide the body with adequate amounts of oxygen and nutrients.

However, scientists are finding new and innovative ways to prevent and treat heart failure. Perhaps the most significant contribution to this effort is the angiotensin-converting enzyme (ACE) inhibitor, a drug that relaxes constricted blood vessels.

Read on for information on these and other medications.

How much is 2,000 gallons?
Enough to fill four large hot tubs

Flush a toilet 1,000 times

Fill your car's gas tank 125 times

Abnormal heart rhythm

Abnormal heart rhythm is also known as **arrhythmia** or irregular heartbeat. It comes in two major forms: tachycardia (abnormally rapid heartbeat) and bradycardia (abnormally slow heartbeat). Isolated instances of arrhythmia are common and usually harmless.

Symptoms of tachycardia: feeling of the heartbeat (palpitations), chest discomfort, weakness, fainting, sweating, shortness of breath, confusion, or dizziness.

Symptoms of bradycardia: fatigue, shortness of breath, lightheadedness, and fainting.

There are two main types of tachycardia. When the upper chambers of the heart beat too fast or irregularly, this is called **atrial fibrillation**. Some drugs are used either to prevent atrial fibrillation from occurring or to prevent the rapid heartbeat from spreading to the lower chambers of the heart (the ventricles).

Ventricular arrhythmias occur when the lower chambers of the heart beat irregularly or add or miss beats. Since the ventricles are responsible for most of the pumping of the heart, it is much more important that persistent ventricular arrhythmias be treated.

How heart drugs help

- Diuretics relieve water retention
- Digitalis drugs help the heart beat stronger and/or control heart rate
- Beta blockers prevent the heart from working too hard
- Calcium channel blockers dilate the arteries and lower blood pressure
- Nitrates dilate the blood vessels
- Lipid-lowering drugs lower cholesterol in various ways

STOP **General Warnings**

- **If scheduled for surgery, make sure to tell your surgeon or anesthesiologist that you are taking these drugs.**
- **Do not use herbal medications for an extended period of time.**

There is no human activity, eating, sleeping, drinking, or sex, which some doctor somewhere won't discover leads directly to cardiac arrest.

JOHN MORTIMER

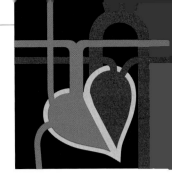

Common drugs for abnormal heart rhythm

Report any side effects to doctor if severe or persistent. Those in orange, *report immediately.*

Important side effects	Negative drug interactions	Special warnings

Mexitil *(mexiletine),* an antiarrhythmic $$

Dizziness, lightheadedness, nausea, vomiting, abdominal pain, heartburn, nervousness, unsteadiness, difficulty walking, trembling, chest pain, heartbeat changes, shortness of breath, convulsions, bleeding, bruising, fever, chills	*Use caution with:* alcohol, antacids, caffeine, other antiarrhythmics (Inderal, Norpace, Quinidex), digitalis preparations (Cedilanid-D, Crystodigin, Lanoxin), Dilantin *(phenytoin),* diuretics (Bumex, Diuril, Diamox), *phenobarbital,* Rifadin *(rifampin),* potassium, Tagamet *(cimetidine),* and *theophylline.*	*Do not use if:* you have severe heart block. *Use caution if:* you've had a bad reaction to other antiarrhythmic drugs or have liver problems, Parkinson's disease, a history of heart disease, low blood pressure, or seizure disorders. Evaluation of heart function is needed before and during use of Mexitil.

Norpace *(disopyramide),* an antiarrhythmic $

Dizziness, faintness, weakness, blurred vision, constipation, dry eyes, mouth or nose, chest pain, shortness of breath, heartbeat changes, fainting, weight gain, swelling of fingers or ankles, anxiety	*Do not combine with:* alcohol and other antiarrhthmics (Inderal, Norpace, Quinidex). *Use caution with:* digitalis preparations (Cedilanid-D, Crystodigin, Lanoxin), Dilantin *(phenytoin),* diuretics (Bumex, Diuril, Diamox), drugs that inhibit the breakdown of other drugs by the liver, *erythromycin,* and other heart regulation medications.	*Do not use if:* you have severe or bifasicular heart block, sick sinus syndrome, or are in heart shock. *Use caution if:* you've had a bad reaction to an antiarrhythmic drug; have heart disease, kidney or liver problems, glaucoma, or an enlarged prostate; or a history of atrial fibrillation, low blood potassium, low blood pressure, low white blood cells, glaucoma, myasthenia gravis, or low blood sugar. Evaluation of heart function is needed before and during use of Norpace.

Procan SR *(procainamide),* an antiarrhythmic $$$

Diarrhea, abdominal pain, nausea, vomiting, appetite loss, fainting, heartbeat changes, fever, chills, joint pain or swelling, painful	*Use caution with:* alcohol, antiarrhthmics (Inderal, Norpace, Quinidex), Cordarone *(amiodarone),* digitalis preparations (Cedilanid-D,	*Do not use if:* you have severe heart block, systemic lupus erythematosus, or myasthenia gravis.

continued on next page

Common drugs for abnormal heart rhythm *continued*

Important side effects	Negative drug interactions	Special warnings

Procan SR *continued*

breathing, rash, itching, confusion, sore mouth, gums or throat, hallucinations, depression, bleeding, bruising, fatigue	Crystodigin, Lanoxin), diuretics (Bumex, Diuril, Diamox), drugs that ease muscle spasms, Proloprim *(trimethoprim)*, Tagamet *(cimetidine)*, and Zantac *(ranitidine)*.	*Use caution if:* you are allergic to local anesthetics with "cain" in their names; have liver or kidney problems, or an enlarged prostate; have a history of heart disease, low blood pressure, abnormally low blood platelet counts; or will have surgery in the near future.

⚠ Quinidex Extentabs *(quinidine)*, an antiarrhythmic $$

Diarrhea occurs in up to 30% of patients. Other side effects include appetite loss, bitter taste, flushing and itching skin, nausea, vomiting, stomach pain or cramps, dizziness, lightheadedness, fainting, vision changes, fever, headache, buzzing in ears, hearing loss, rash, hives, shortness of breath, wheezing, rapid heartbeat, bleeding, bruising, fatigue	*Do not combine with:* Norvir *(ritonavir)* and tobacco. *Use caution with:* antacids containing magnesium, antidepressants (Elavil, Nardil, Prozac), antiarrythmics (Cordarone, Mexitil, Norpace, Procanbid), antispasmodics (Banthine, Darbid, Pro-Banthine), aspirin, beta blockers (Inderal, Sectral, Tenormin), calcium channel blockers (Calan, Cardene, Procardia), Carafate *(sucralfate)*, codeine, Coumadin *(warfarin)*, Crystodigin *(digitoxin)*, Dilantin *(phenytoin)*, diuretics (Bumex, Diuril, Diamox), Haldol *(haloperidol)*, Lanoxin *(digoxin)*, Nizoral *(ketoconazole)*, phenobarbital, phenothiazines (Serentine, Stelazine, Thorazine), Rifadin *(rifampin)*, sodium bicarbonate, Tagamet *(cimetidine)*, and Vicodin *(hydrocodone)*.	*Do not use if:* you have an infection, myasthenia gravis, abnormal heart rhythms, or have taken too much Lanoxin *(digoxin)*. *Use caution if:* you have liver problems, coronary artery disease, low blood pressure, acute rheumatic fever, subacute bacterial endocarditis, a history of hyperthyroidism or blood platelet deficiency, or will have surgery in the near future.

⚠ Sectral *(acebutolol)*, a beta blocker $$$

Cough, diarrhea, decreased libido, depression, drowsiness, dizziness, fatigue, frequent urination, gas, indigestion, nausea, trouble sleeping, cold hands and feet, numbness or tingling in fingers or toes, shortness of breath, rapid heartbeat, worsening of asthma, rash, itching, wheezing, swelling of lips, tongue and throat	*Do not take with:* Mao inhibitors (Marplan, Nardil, Parnate). Wait at least two weeks after your last dose before taking Sectral. *Use caution with:* albuterol, Alazine *(hydralazine)*, calcium channel blockers (Adalat CC, Cardizem, Norvasc), certain blood pressure medications, certain over-the-counter cold remedies and nasal drops, Cordarone *(amiodarone)*,	*Do not use if:* you are in heart failure, if you have severe heart block or a slow heart rate. *Use caution if:* you've had a bad reaction to beta blockers; have heart disease, heart failure, hay fever, asthma, chronic bronchitis, emphysema, hyperthyroidism, liver or kidney problems, diabetes, or myasthenia gravis; have a history of low blood sugar; suffer

56

continued on next page

Chapter **4**

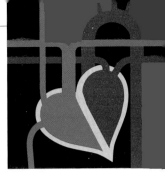

Important side effects	Negative drug interactions	Special warnings

Common drugs for abnormal heart rhythm *continued*

Sectral *continued*

| | digitalis (Cedilanid-D, Crystodigin, Lanoxin), Effexor *(venlafaxine)*, nasal deconges- tants, nonsteroidal anti- inflammatories (Aleve, Daypro, Indocin, Toradol), Norpace *di*oral antidiabetics (Amaryl, Glucotrol, Micronase), *quinidine*, and reserpine | from problems with circulation to the arms and legs; or will have surgery in the near future. Never stop Sectral suddenly without help from your doctor. |

Tenormin *(atenolol)*, a beta blocker $

| Decreased libido, decreased mobility, dizziness, lighthead- edness, drowsiness, fatigue, weakness, insomnia, depres- sion, shortness of breath, wheezing, slow heartbeat, chest pain or tightness, swelling of ankles, feet and lower legs | *Use caution with:* ampicillin, calcium channel blockers (Adalat CC, Cardizem, Norvasc), calcium-containing antacids, Catapres *(cloni- dine)*, certain blood pressure medications, digitalis, EdiPen *(epinephrine)*, insulin, oral antidiabetics (Amaryl, Glucotrol, Micronase), *peni- cillin*, Quinidex *(quinidine)*, and reserpine. | *Do not use if:* you are in heart failure or cardiogenic shock, have severe heart block, a slow heart rate, or have taken an MAO inhibitor antidepres- sant (Nardil) in the past 14 days. *Use caution if:* you have had a bad reaction to beta blockers, have low blood pressure, liver or kidney problems, diabetes or myasthenia gravis, heart disease, hay fever, asthma, chronic bronchitis, chronic obstructive pulmonary dis- ease, emphysema, hyperthy- roidism, or will have surgery in the near future. Do not stop Tenormin suddenly without help from your doctor. |

Lily of the Valley

| Large amounts can cause nausea, vomiting, headache, stupor, disorders of color per- ception, irregular heartbeat | *Use caution with:* calcium, lax- atives, glucocorticoids, *quini- dine* (Quinaglute), saluretics, steroid medications, and water pills (Lasix). | |

Mate

| Large amounts can cause restlessness, irritability, insomnia, palpitations, dizzi- ness, vomiting, diarrhea, loss of appetite, headache. | | *Do not use if:* you are sensitive to caffeine. |

Angina

Angina pain is caused when the heart muscle is not getting enough oxygen.

Symptoms: a squeezing or pressure-like pain in the chest, usually after exertion, although it can sometimes happen at rest. The pain may extend to the left shoulder blade, left arm or jaw, and usually lasts up to 20 minutes. Some of the drugs below are used to treat or prevent the pain of angina. Other drugs are used to prevent heart attack, since angina increases the risk of heart attack.

If you are a man over the age of 50, ask your doctor whether you should be taking small doses of aspirin every day. Aspirin has been shown to decrease the likelihood of men over age 50 to have a first heart attack, and it decreases the number of men and women who already have had a heart attack from having a second one.

Common drugs for angina

Report any side effects to doctor if severe or persistent. Those in orange, report immediately.

Important side effects	Negative drug interactions	Special warnings
Cardizem *(diltiazem)*, a calcium channel blocker		**$$$**
Swelling, headache, flushing , dizziness, drowsiness, constipation, nausea, weight gain, fatigue, heartbeat changes, shortness of breath	*Use caution with:* beta blockers (Inderal, Sectral, Tenormin), *cyclosporine, digitalis*, Lanoxin *(digoxin)*, Tagamet *(cimetidine)*, and Tegretol *(carbamazepine)*.	*Do not use if:* you have sick sinus syndrome, second- or third-degree heart block, low blood pressure, or heart failure. *Use caution if:* you have had a bad reaction to a calcium blocker, have liver or kidney problems, or a history of congestive heart failure.
Imdur *(isosorbide mononitrate)*, a nitrate		**$$$**
Dizziness, lightheadedness, flushing of face and neck, rapid pulse or heartbeat, nausea, vomiting, restlessness, blurred vision, dry mouth, headache	*Do not combine with:* alcohol, tobacco, and Viagra *(sildenafil)*. *Use caution with:* alcohol or calcium-blocking blood pressure medications (Calan, Cardizem, Procardia).	*Do not use if:* you have had a recent heart attack or have high blood pressure, tachycardia, congestive heart failure, severe anemia, hyperthyroidism, or a hypertrophic cardiomyopathy. *Use caution if:* you have had a bad reaction to other nitrate drugs or vasodilators, have had a cerebral hemorrhage recently, have glaucoma, or a history of low blood pressure. Report any severe or prolonged headaches.

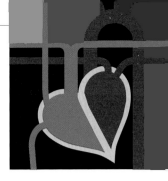

Common drugs for angina *continued*

Important side effects	Negative drug interactions	Special warnings

Nitrostat *(nitroglycerin)*, a nitrate $

Flushing of face and neck, headache, nausea, vomiting, dizziness, lightheadedness, rapid heartbeat, restlessness, blurred vision, rash, dry mouth	*Do not combine with:* alcohol and Viagra *(sildenafil).* *Use caution with:* aspirin, beta blockers (Inderal, Sectral, Tenormin), blood vessel dilators, calcium channel blockers (Adalat CC, Cardizem, Norvasc), *dihydroergotamine,* high blood pressure medications, *isosorbide dinitrate,* and *isosorbide mononitrate.*	*Use caution if:* you have had a bad reaction to other nitrates, have low blood pressure, problems absorbing medicine, excessive stomach action, or bleeding in your head. Report any severe or prolonged headaches.

Norvasc *(amlodipine)*—see high blood pressure (hypertension)

Procardia XL *(nifedipine)*—see high blood pressure

verapamil, a calcium channel blocker $$

Constipation, headache, dizziness, flushing, feeling of warmth, swelling in feet, ankles and calves, palpitations, breathing difficulty, coughing, wheezing, irregular heartbeat, chest pain, extreme dizziness, and fainting	*Do not combine with:* grapefruit juice or grapefruit. *Use caution with:* anti-arrhythmics (Cordarone, Norpace, *quinidine,* Tambocor), beta blockers (Inderal, Sectral, Tenormin), *cyclosporine,* Dilantin *(phenytoin),* diuretics, Glucotrol *(glipizide),* high blood pressure drugs, Lanoxin *(digitalis),* Lithonate *(lithium),* nitrates, *phenobarbital,* Rifadin *(rifampin),* Tagamet *(cimetidine),* Tegretol *(carbamazepine),* Theo-Dur *(theophylline),* Tofranil *(imipramine).*	*Do not use if:* you have liver disease, a sick sinus syndrome, a fast heart rate, second- or third-degree heart block, low blood pressure, or advanced aortic stenosis. *Use caution if:* you have had a bad reaction to a calcium channel blocker; have poor circulation to the extremities; suffer from gangrene, liver, or kidney problems; have a history of congestive heart failure, abnormal heart rhythm, drug-induced liver damage; or have had a recent stroke or heart attack. If angina gets worse, call your doctor immediately.

Hawthorn leaf

Congestive heart failure

Congestive heart failure refers to an inability of the heart to pump enough blood effectively.

Symptoms: weakness, fatigue and shortness of breath, lower extremity swelling.

Common drugs for congestive heart failure

Report any side effects to doctor if severe or persistent. Those in orange, report immediately.

Important side effects	Negative drug interactions	Special warnings
Accupril *(quinapril)*—see high blood pressure (hypertension)		
Altace *(ramipril)*—see high blood pressure		
Capoten *(captopril)*—see high blood pressure		
Lotensin *(benazepril)*—see high blood pressure		
Mavik *(trandolapril)*—see high blood pressure		
Monopril *(fosinopril)*—see high blood pressure		
Prinivil *(lisinopril)*—see high blood pressure		
Univasc *(moexipril)*—see high blood pressure		
Vasotec *(enalapril)*—see high blood pressure		
Zestril *(lisinopril)*—see high blood pressure		

Coreg *(carvedilol)*, a beta blocker $$$$$

Important side effects	Negative drug interactions	Special warnings
Dizziness, lightheadedness, decreased sexual ability, fatigue, weakness, drowsiness, insomnia; diarrhea, nausea, vomiting, shortness of breath, wheezing, irregular or slow heartbeat (50 beats per minute or less), pain, pressure or tightness in chest, swelling of ankles, feet, and lower legs, or depression	*Use caution with:* amphetamines, oral antidiabetic agents, insulin, asthma medication (such as *aminophylline* or *theophylline*), calcium channel blockers, *clonidine, guanabenz,* immunotherapy for allergies (allergy shots), MAO inhibitors, *reserpine,* or other beta blockers. Coreg interacts with many over-the-counter medicines.	*Use caution if:* you have allergies, asthma; diabetes, heart or blood vessel disease (including peripheral vascular disease), hyperthyroidism, or irregular (slow) heartbeat; a history of mental depression; myasthenia gravis, psoriasis, or respiratory problems such as bronchitis or emphysema; or kidney or liver disease. Those over 60 should have smaller doses and frequent blood pressure checks.

furosemide, a loop diuretic $

Important side effects	Negative drug interactions	Special warnings
Muscle cramps, weakness, or pain, heart palpitations, weakness, dizziness, thirst, dry mouth, constipation, rash, hives, itching, swelling of mouth and throat, breathing difficulty, mood changes, nausea, vomiting, fatigue, black or tarry stools	*Use caution with:* Atromid-S *(clofibrate),* Colestid *(colestipol),* cortisone, digitalis preparations, Dilantin *(phenytoin),* high blood pressure medications, Indocin *(indomethacin),* Lithonate *(lithium),* nonsteroidal anti-inflammatory drugs, oral antidiabetics (Amaryl, Glucotrol, Micronase), Paxil *(paroxetine),* phenobarbital,	*Do not use if:* your kidneys are not making urine. *Use caution if:* you are allergic to any "sulfa" drug; have diabetes, gout, lupus erythematosus, impaired hearing, or low blood potassium or other electrolytes; have a history of liver or kidney disease; or will have surgery in the near future.

continued on next page

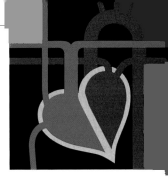

Common drugs for congestive heart failure *continued*

Important side effects	Negative drug interactions	Special warnings
furosemide *continued*		
	Prozac *(fluoxetine)*, Questran *(cholestyramine)*, salicylates, Vasotec *(enalapril)*, and Zoloft *(sertraline)*.	Take *furosemide* one hour before or two hours after meals.

Lasix *(furosemide)*, a loop diuretic $

Muscle cramps or pain, heartbeat changes, weakness, dizziness, thirst, dry mouth, constipation, rash, hives, itching, swelling of mouth and throat, breathing difficulty, lightheadedness, bleeding, bruising	*Use caution with:* all antidiabetcs (Amaryl, *insulin*, Micronase), barbiturates (Amytal, Seconal, Solfoton), Colestid *(colestipol)*, corticosteroids, *digitalis*, high blood pressure medications, Lanoxin *(digoxin)*, Lithonate *(lithium)*, nonsteroidal anti-inflammatories (Aleve, Daypro, Toradol), Mexate *(methotrexate)*, and Questran *(cholestyramine)*.	*Do not use if:* your kidneys are not making urine or have severe congestive heart failure. *Use with caution if:* you are allergic to sulfa drugs, other medicines, or the dye tartrazine; have asthma, diabetes, gout, or lupus erythematosus; have history of kidney or liver diease or pancreatitis; have had electrolyte tests your doctor has not seen; or will will have surgery in the near future. This drug can lead to decreased levels of blood potassium and magnesium; you may need to supplement your diet.

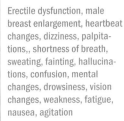

Lanoxin *(digoxin)*, a digitalis drug $

Erectile dysfunction, male breast enlargement, heartbeat changes, dizziness, palpitations,, shortness of breath, sweating, fainting, hallucinations, confusion, mental changes, drowsiness, vision changes, weakness, fatigue, nausea, agitation	*Use caution with:* Aldactone *(spironolactone)*, all nonprescription medications, antacids, antiarrythmics (Inderal, Norpace, Quinidex, Rythmol), beta blockers (Inderal, Sectral, Tenormin), Azulfidine *(sulfasalazine)*, calcium channel blockers (Adalat CC, Cardizem, Norvasc), Carafate *(sucralfate)*, certain anticancer medications, including Neosar *(cyclophosphamide)*, Colestid *(colestipol)*, diuretics (Bumex, Diuril, Diamox), Indocin *(indomethacin)*, kaolin-pectin, Midamor *(amiolride)*, Norpace *(disopyramide)*, over-the-counter cold, cough, or allergy	*Use caution if:* you have had a bad reaction to digitalis; have taken digitalis or a diuretic in the past 14 days; have abnormal heart rhythms, aortic problems, damage to the heart muscle, liver or kidney problems, a history of lung disease, low blood potassium or magnesium, or thyroid function disorder. Avoid excessive caffeine.

continued on next page

Common drugs for congestive heart failure *continued*

Important side effects	Negative drug interactions	Special warnings

Lanoxin *continued*

	remedies, Questran *(choles-tyramine)*, Reglan *(metoclo-pramide)*, Rifadin *(rifampin)*, Sandimmune *(cyclosporine)*, Sporanox *(itraconazole)*, steroids, thyroid hormones (Cytomel, Synthroid), water pills, and Xanax *(alprazolam)*.	

Zaroxolyn *(metolazone)*, a thiazide diuretic $$

Weakness, dizziness, thirst, dry mouth, constipation, skin rash, hives, intense itching, swelling of the mouth and throat, breathing difficulty, heart rhythm irregularities, lightheadedness, unusual bleeding or bruising, severe dehydration	*Use caution with:* anticoagulants, all antidiabetcs (Amaryl, *insulin,* Micronase), barbiturates (Amytal, Seconal, Solfoton), Colestid *(colestipol)*, corticosteroids, digitalis, high blood pressure medications, Lanoxin *(digoxin)*, Lithonate *(lithium)*, nonsteroidal anti-inflammatories (Aleve, Daypro, Toradol), Mexate *(methotrexate)*, and Questran *(cholestyramine)*.	*Do not use if:* your kidneys are not making urine. *Use caution if:* you have diabetes, gout, lupus erythematosus, pancreatitis, heart disease, blood vessel disease, liver disease, or kidney disease or have had allergic reactions to metolazone, carbonic anhydrase inhibitors like *acetazolamide,* sulfa drugs, foods, dyes, or preservatives.

K-Dur, potassium supplement
Slow-K, potassium supplement
Micro-K, potassium supplement
Klor-kon, potassium supplement
K-tab, potassium supplement
potassium chloride, potassium supplement

Numbness or tingling in hands, feet or lips, irregular heartbeat, breathing difficulty, fatigue, weakness, confusion, diarrhea, abdominal discomfort, gas, nausea, vomiting	*Do not use with:* ACE inhibitors (Altace, Capoten, Vasotec), antacids, potassium-sparing diuretics (Aldactone, Dyazide, Maxzide, Moduretic), salt substitutes. *Use caution with:* beta blockers (Inderal, Tenormin, Toprol), Lanoxin *(digoxin)*, *lithium,* nonsteroidal anti-inflammatories.	

Lipitor versus angioplasty

Lipitor is at least as effective as angioplasty for patients with mild coronary artery disease, according to a study in **The New England Journal of Medicine** sponsored by its manufacturer **Warner-Lambert.** The 341 study participants were all slated for angioplasty. Half got Lipitor instead, and the remaining patients underwent angioplasty followed by "usual care, which could include lipid-lowering treatment." After 18 months, 21% of the angioplasty patients had had heart attacks, compared with only 13% of those on Lipitor.

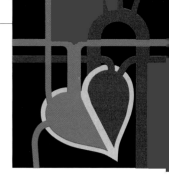

High cholesterol

Cholesterol is a naturally occurring fat, and the liver makes all the cholesterol the body normally needs. Elevated blood cholesterol levels and high triglycerides are risk factors for heart disease. (Smoking, however, is a ten-fold higher risk.)

Common drugs for high cholesterol and high triglycerides

Report any side effects to doctor if severe or persistent. Those in orange, report immediately.

Important side effects	Negative drug interactions	Special warnings
Baycol *(cerivastatin)*, an antihyperlipidemic		**$$$$**
Muscle pain, tenderness or weakness, exhaustion, fever, abdominal pain, swelling, chest pain, rash, constipation, diarrhea, nausea, gas, indigestion, heartburn, insomnia	*Use caution with:* alcohol, antifungals, *erythromycin, gemfibrozil,* immunosuppressants, Niacin *(nicotinic acid),* over-the-counter medications.	*Use caution if:* you abuse alcohol, if you have any allergies, liver disease, high levels of liver enzymes, seizures, electrolyte disorders, severe infection, low blood pressure, or if you have had recent surgery or trauma.
Lescol *(fluvastatin)*, an antilipidemic (cholesterol-lowering agent)		**$$$**
Headache, dyspepsia, back pain, upper respiratory tract infection, influenza, constipation, diarrhea, dizziness, lightheadedness, bloating, gas, heartburn, nausea, rash, stomach pain, fever, muscle pain	*Use caution with:* Coumadin *(warfarin),* digoxin, erythromycin, Lopid *(gemfibrozil),* Nizoral *(ketoconazole),* Questran *(cholestyramine),* and Rifadin *(rifampin).*	*Do not use if:* you have liver disease. *Use caution if:* you have previously taken a cholesterol-reducing drug; have cataracts, impaired vision, chronic muscle disorder, a history of liver problems, drink a lot of alcohol, or plan major surgery in the near future. Periodic eye exams may be necessary.
Lipitor *(atorvastatin)*, an antilipidemic		**$$$$**
Headache, myalgia, diarrhea, constipation, dizziness, lightheadedness, bloating, gas, heartburn, nausea, rash, stomach pain, fever, unexplained muscle aches and tenderness, vision changes	*Use caution with:* Calan *(verapamil),* cyclosporine, Lanoxin *(digoxin),* Diflucan *(fluconazole), erythromycin,* grapefruit juice, Lopid *(gemfibrizil),* niacin, Nizoral *(ketoconazole),* oral contraceptives (Loestrin, Nordette, Ortho Cyclen), and Sporanox *(itraconazole).*	*Do not use if:* you have unexplained increased liver function tests or liver disease. *Use caution if:* you have previously taken a cholesterol-lowering drug or have liver problems, kidney disease, chronic muscle disorder, drink a lot of alcohol, or will have major surgery in the near future. Periodic eye exams may be needed.

Common drugs for high cholesterol and high triglycerides *continued*

Important side effects	Negative drug interactions	Special warnings

Lopid *(gemfibrozil)*, an antilipidemic $

Diarrhea, nausea, muscle aches and tenderness, abdominal pain, nausea, vomiting, decreased urination, signs of infection	*Use caution with:* anticoagulants, *colestipol, gylburide, lovastatin,* and *pravastatin.*	*Do not use if:* you have biliary cirrhosis of the liver or kidney problems. *Use caution if:* you have liver or kidney problems, gallbladder disease, gallstones, diabetes, or hypothyroidism. Inform your doctor if you have used *clofibrate* in the past. Periodic triglyceride and cholesterol levels are critical.

Mevacor *(lovastatin)*, an antilipidemic $$$

Headache, diarrhea, constipation, flatulence, rash , abdominal pain, nausea, dizziness, blurred vision, lightheadedness, bloating, gas, heartburn, stomach pain, fever, unexplained muscle aches and tenderness	*Do not combine with:* Atromid-S *(clofibrate),* Calan *(verapamil),* Diflucan *(fluconazole),* grapefruit juice, Lopid *(gemfibrozil),* Nizoral *(ketoconazole),* Serzone *(nefazodone),* Sporanox *(itraconazole).* *Use caution with:* Biaxin *(clarithromycin),* Cardizem *(diltiazem),* Coumadin *(warfarin),* cyclosporine, and other immunosuppressive drugs, *erythromycin,* Lamisil *(terbinafine), niacin,* and *nicotinic acid.*	*Do not use if:* you have liver disease. *Use caution if:* you have liver problems, peptic ulcer disease, upper gastrointestinal bleeding, cataracts, chronic muscle disorder, impaired vision, a history of kidney problems, drink a lot of alcohol, or will have surgery in the near future. Periodic eye exams may be needed.

Pravachol *(pravastatin)*, an antilipidemic $$

Headache, diarrhea, constipation, flatulence, rash, abdominal pain, nausea and vomiting, localized pain, cold, dizziness, blurred vision, lightheadedness, bloating, gas, heartburn, stomach pain, fever, unexplained muscle aches and tenderness, vision changes	*Do not use with:* grapefruit juice. *Use caution with:* Colestid *(colestipol),* Coumadin *(warfarin),* drugs that suppress the immune system, *erythromycin,* Lopid *(gemfibrozil), niacin,* Nizoral *(ketoconazole),* Questran *(cholestyramine),* Serzone *(nefazodone),* and Tagamet *(cimetidine).*	*Do not use if:* you have liver disease. *Use caution if:* you have previously taken a cholesterol-lowering drug, have kidney disease, cataracts, impaired vision, chronic muscle disorder, a history of liver problems, drink a lot of alcohol, or will have surgery in the near future. Periodic eye exams may be needed.

Tricor *(fenofibrate)*, an antihyperlipidemic $$$

Muscle pain, tenderness or weakness, exhaustion, fever, sore throat, chills, nausea, vomiting, itching, skin rash	*Use caution with:* anticoagulants *(dicumarol,* Miradon, *warfarin),* cyclosporine, and statin drugs.	*Use caution if:* you have gallbladder disease, gallstones, liver or kidney disease.

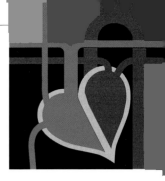

Important side effects	Negative drug interactions	Special warnings
Zocor *(simvastatin)*, an antilipidemic		**$$**
Frequent urge to urinate, nervousness, restlessness, mental changes, muscle twitching or pain, nausea, vomiting, slow breathing, headache, appetite loss, swelling of feet or lower legs, bad taste, fatigue, vision changes	*Do not use with:* Calan *(verapamil)*, Cardizem *(diltiazem)*, erythromycin, grapefruit juice, Lopid *(gemfibrozil)*, Nizoral *(ketoconazole)*, Prozac *(fluoxetine)*, and Serzone *(nefazodone)*. *Use caution with:* Biaxin *(clarithromycin), cyclosporine, digoxin, nicotinic acid,* Posicor *(mibefradil),* and Questran *(cholestyramine).*	*Do not use if:* you have liver disease. *Use caution if:* you have previously taken a cholesterol-lowering medication, or if you have cataracts, chronic muscle disorder, or impaired vision, a history of liver problems, drink a lot of alcohol, or will have surgery in the near future. Periodic eye exams may be needed.
Fo-ti		
Diarrhea, flushing of the face, digestive distress		*Do not use if:* you have phlegm or diarrhea.
Psyllium		
Runny nose, pinkeye, asthma, hives	Wait at least one hour after taking any other medications before taking psyllium.	*Do not use if:* you have a bowel obstruction, diabetes, or a narrowing of the digestive tract. Take psyllium with plenty of water.
Soy lecithin		
Mild digestive upset, including stomach pain, loose stools, diarrhea		
Garlic		
Nausea, stomach complaints		*Use caution if:* you are taking blood thinners.
Wild yam		

Common drugs for high cholesterol and high triglycerides *continued*

Neglected Statins

The cholesterol-lowering **statins**—Lipitor *(atorvastatin)*, Zocor *(simvastatin)*, Pravachol *(pravastatin)*, Lescol *(fluvastatin)*, Mevacor *(lovastatin)* and Baycol *(cerivastatin)*—are easy to take, have relatively few side effects, and have dropped cholesterol levels by 60 points, but few take them. About 8 million Americans take them, while experts estimate that 20 to 30 million would benefit from them.

High blood pressure (hypertension)

Blood pressure refers to the resistance produced each time the heart beats and sends blood through the arteries. High blood pressure (also known as hypertension) is a major risk factor for heart attack and stroke. It is divided into four categories: borderline, mild, moderate, and severe.

Common drugs for high blood pressure

Report any side effects to doctor if severe or persistent. Those in orange, report immediately.

Important side effects	Negative drug interactions	Special warnings
Adalat CC (*nifedipine*), a calcium channel blocker		$$$
Procardia XL (nifedipine), a calcium channel blocker		$$$$
Peripheral swelling, dizziness , headache, weakness, nausea, palpitations, nervousness, pulmonary edema, congestive heart failure, myocardial infarction, skin flushing and feeling of warmth, swelling in feet, ankles or calves, palpitations, breathing difficulty, coughing, wheezing, irregular heartbeat, chest pain, fainting, skin problems, changes in thirst or urination	*Do not combine with:* alcohol or grapefruit juice. *Use caution with:* anti-arrhythmics, beta blockers (Inderal, Sectral, Tenormin), drugs that lower blood pressure, Lanoxin (*digoxin*), *quinidine,* Tagamet (*cimetidine),* and Zantac (*ranitidine*).	*Do not use if:* you have liver disease, low blood pressure, narrowing of the aorta, or if you are over 70 and have been prescribed the immediate-release form of nifedipine. *Use caution if:* you have had a bad reaction to calcium channel blockers; have cardiomyopathy, kidney problems, atrial fibrillation, diabetes, abnormal heart rhythm, or Duchenne muscular dystrophy; or have a history of congestive heart failure, heart attack, stroke, or drug-induced liver damage. Call your doctor if you have angina and it worsens. Carry a card stating that you are taking Procardia.
Accupril (*quinapril*), angiotensin-converting enzyme (ACE) inhibitor		$$$
Altace (*ramipril*), angiotensin-converting enzyme (ACE) inhibitor		$$$
Capoten (*captopril*), angiotensin-converting enzyme (ACE) inhibitor		$
Lotensin (*benazepril*), angiotensin-converting enzyme (ACE) inhibitor		$$
Mavik (*trandolapril*), angiotensin-converting enzyme (ACE) inhibitor		$$
Monopril (*fosinopril*), angiotensin-converting enzyme (ACE) inhibitor		$$
Prinivil (*lisinopril*), angiotensin-converting enzyme (ACE) inhibitor		$$
Univasc (*moexipril*), angiotensin-converting enzyme (ACE) inhibitor		$$

continued on next page

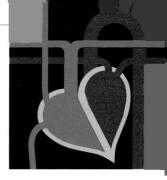

Common drugs for high-blood pressure *continued*

Important side effects	Negative drug interactions	Special warnings

Zestril *(lisinopril),* angiotensin-converting enzyme (ACE) inhibitor $$

Important side effects	Negative drug interactions	Special warnings
Dry cough, fever, chills, sore throat hoarseness, difficulty breathing or swallowing, swelling of face, mouth or extremities, ankle swelling, decreased urination, confusion, discoloration of eyes or skin, itching, chest pain palpitations, abdominal pain, weight gain	*Use caution with:* antihypertensives (Cardura, Catapres, Lotensin), diuretics (Bumex. Diuril, Diamox), Indocin *(indomethacin), lithium,* nitrates, potassium-containing salt substitutes, potassium-sparing diuretics (Aldactazide, Moduretic), potassium supplements, and Zyloprim *(allopurinol).*	*Do not use if:* you have a blood cell or bone marrow disorder, or an abnormally high level of potassium. *Use caution if:* you have kidney problems, scleroderma, systemic lupus erythematosus, heart or liver disease, diabetes, renal artery stenosis, or will have surgery in the near future. Report signs of infection or water retention. Blood counts and urine analyses are needed before use of these drugs. Do not take potassium supplements with these drugs.

Cardene *(nicardipine),* calcium channel blocker and antihypertensive $$$$

Norvasc *(amlodipine),* calcium channel blocker and antihypertensive $$$

Plendil *(felodipine),* calcium channel blocker and antihypertensive $$

Important side effects	Negative drug interactions	Special warnings
Headache, peripheral swelling, flushing in face and body, decreased urination, swelling of feet and ankles, weight gain, increased angina attacks, dizziness upon arising from a sitting or lying position, shortness of breath, weakness, slow heartbeat, rash	*Do not use with*: grapefruit juice. *Use caution with:* alcohol, azole antifungals (e.g., Diflucan, Nizoral, Sporanox), beta blockers (Inderal, Sectral, Tenormin), digitalis preparations, drugs that lower blood pressure, Norvir *(ritonavir),* Rescriptor *(delavirdine),* and Sandimmune *(cyclosporine).*	*Do not use if:* you have liver disease, low blood pressure, atrioventricular block, sick sinus syndrome, or a dysfunctional left heart ventricle. *Use caution if:* you have had a bad reaction to calcium blockers, or if you have congestive heart failure, heart attack, stroke, abnormal heart rhythm, circulation problems in your hands, muscular dystrophy, or a history of drug-induced liver damage. Carry a card stating that you are taking Norvasc. Call your doctor if you have angina and it gets worse.

Common drugs for high-blood pressure *continued*

Important side effects	Negative drug interactions	Special warnings

Cardizem—see angina

Flomax *(tamsulosin)*—see prostate problems
Hytrin *(terazosin)*—see prostate problems

Dizziness, headache, nasal congestion, asthenia, peripheral swelling, drowsiness, chest pain	**Do not combine with:** tobacco. **Use caution with:** nonprescription medications for allergic rhinitis or colds, nonsteroidal anti-inflammatories (Aleve, Daypro, Toradol), and other blood pressure drugs.	**Do not use if:** you have mental depression or angina. **Use caution if:** you have light-headedness upon standing, impaired circulation to the brain, coronary artery disease, liver or kidney problems, a history of mental depression or stroke, or will have surgery in the near future. Use caution when operating heavy machinery while taking Hytrin.

Lopressor *(metoprolol)*, beta-blocker — $
Sectral *(acebutolol)*, beta-blocker — $$$
Tenormin *(atenolol)*, beta-blocker — $
Toprol *(metoprolol)*, beta-blocker — $$

Dizziness, lightheadedness, decreased sexual ability, fatigue, weakness, drowsiness, insomnia, shortness of breath, wheezing, irregular or slow heartbeat, chest pain or tightness, swelling of ankles, feet and lower legs, depression	**Use caution with:** Brethine *(terbutaline)*, Apresoline *(hydralazine)*, barbiturates (Amytal, *phenobarbital*, Seconal,), calcium channel blockers (Calan, Cardizem, Norvasc), Catapres *(clonidine)*, Cipro *(ciprofloxacin)*, Cordarone *(amiodarone)*, drugs to lower blood pressure, EpiPen *(epinephrine)*, Minipress *(prazosin)*, nonsteroidal anti-inflammatories (Aleve, Daypro, Naprosyn), oral antidiabetics (Avandia, Glucophage, Glucotrol), Quinaglute *(quinidine)*, reserpine, Rifadin *(rifampin)*, Tagamet *(cimetidine)*, and Zantac *(ranitidine)*.	**Use caution if:** you have trouble with beta blockers; have liver or kidney problems, diabetes, or myasthenia gravis; have a history of heart disease, hay fever, asthma, bronchitis, emphysema, hyperthyroidism, low blood sugar, poor circulation to the extremities, or legs cramps; or will have surgery in the near future. Do not stop this drug abruptly without consulting your doctor.

Triamterene, a potassium-sparing diuretic — $

Rash, hives, lightheadedness, bleeding	**Do not combine with:** potassium supplements, potassium-sparing diuretics, and Sandimmune *(cyclosporine)*. **Use caution with:** ACE inhibitors (Accupril, Capoten, Prinivil), antidiabetics (Amaryl,	**Do not use if:** you have liver or kidney problems or if your blood potassium level is elevated. **Use caution if:** you have diabetes or gout; have a history of liver or kidney disease,

continued on next page

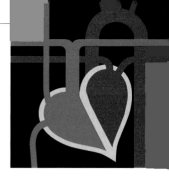

Common drugs for high-blood pressure *continued*		
Important side effects	**Negative drug interactions**	**Special warnings**
Triamterene *continued*		
	insulin, Glucotrol), antigout drugs *(colchicines*, Zyloprim), antihypertensives (Cardura, Catapres, Hytrin), corticosteroids, Coumadin *(warfarin)*, diuretics, laxatives, Lithonate *(lithium)*, nonsteroidal anti-inflammatories (Aleve, Daypro, Toradol), salt substitutes containing potassium, and Urised *(methenamine)*.	G6PD-enzyme deficiency, blood cell disorders; or will have general anestheisa in the near future. Do not consume excessive potassium while taking triamterene. Do not stop this drug abruptly unless high blood levels of potassium develop.
Khella		
Jaundice, queasiness, dizziness, loss of appetite, headache, sleep disorders		Limit exposure to the sun while using khella.
Garlic—see cholesterol		
Kudzu		
Onion		
Stomach irritation		

Some of the hottest heart medications in the U.S.

- Norvasc *(amlopidine)*
  Treats angina and high-blood pressure

- Lanoxin *(digoxin)*
  Treats congestive heart failure and abnormal heart rhythm

- Prinivil *(lisinopril)*
  Zestril *(lisinopril)*
  Treat high blood pressure and advanced heart failure; used to prevent death after heart attacks, treat kidney problems in diabetics, and help prolong life in cases of congestive heart failure

- Vasotec *(enalapril)*
  Treats high blood pressure and advanced heart failure; used to prevent death after heart attacks, treats kidney problems in diabetics, and helps prolong life in cases of congestive heart failure

- Coumadin *(warfarin)*
  Prevents blood clots and pulmonary embolism

- Cardizem *(diltiazem)*
  Treats angina and high-blood pressure

- Lasix *(furosemide)*
  Treats high blood pressure, edema, and heart failure

- Adalat CC
  Procardia XL *(nifedipine)*
  Treats angina and high-blood pressure

- Accupril *(quinapril)*
  Treats high blood pressure and advanced heart failure; used to prevent death after heart attacks, treat kidney problems in diabetics, and help prolong life in cases of congestive heart failure

- Lotensin *(benazepril)*
  Treats high blood pressure and advanced heart failure; used to prevent death after heart attacks, treat kidney problems in diabetics, and help prolong life in cases of congestive heart failure

Stroke

A stroke can occur when the blood supply to the brain is disturbed.

Symptoms: abrupt loss of vision, strength, coordination, sensation, or speech, numbness on one side of the body, sudden and severe headache followed by fainting.

Common drugs for stroke

Report any side effects to doctor if severe or persistent. Those in orange, report immediately.

Important side effects	Negative drug interactions	Special warnings
Coumadin *(warfarin)*, an anticoagulant		**$$**
Bleeding, wheezing, breathing difficulty, hives, swelling of lips, tongue and throat, severe infection, unexpected menstrual bleeding, black vomit, bruises or purple marks on skin	Coumadin interacts with many other medications. Consult your doctor or pharmacist before combining with *any* other prescription drug, non-prescription drug, dietary supplement, or vitamin. *Use caution with:* alcohol and grapefruit juice. Foods high in vitamin K (asparagus, bacon, beef liver, cabbage, fish, cauliflower, green, leafy vegetables) will diminish the effects of the drug.	*Do not use if:* you have a peptic ulcer, ulcerative colitis, arterial aneurysm, low blood platelets, infective pericarditis, liver disease, esophageal varices, or had a recent stroke or spinal anesthesia. *Use caution if:* you have high blood pressure, diabetes, abnormal menstrual bleeding, or impaired liver or kidney function; have a history of bleeding disorders; use an indwelling catheter; or will have surgery or dental extraction in the near future. Always carry a card stating that you are taking Coumadin. Do not change from brand name to generic or vice versa without consulting your doctor.
Plavix *(clopidogrel)*, antiplatelet drug		**$$$$**
Ticlid *(ticlopidine)*, antiplatelet drug		**$$$$$**
Rash, stomach pain, diarrhea, indigestion, nausea, bleeding that is unusually heavy or difficult to stop, bruising, signs of infection, sores, ulcers, white spots in mouth, abdominal pain, back pain, fever, peeling or loosening of skin or lips or mucous membranes, bloody or tarry stools, blood in urine, coughing up blood, dizziness, fever, chills, headache, coordination problems, red spots on skin, thickened or scaly skin, difficulty speaking, vomiting of blood or dark material	*Do not combine with:* anticoagulants, such as Coumadin *(warfarin)*. *Use caution with:* aspirin, cortisone-like drugs, and seizure medications (Depakote, *theophylline*).	*Do not use if:* you have a blood cell, bleeding, or bone marrow disorder, peptic ulcer disease, Crohn's disease, ulcerative colitis, or liver problems. *Use caution if:* you have a history of drug-induced bone marrow depression or blood cell disorder, gastric or duodenal ulcers, kidney problems, or plan to have surgery in the near future. White blood cell counts may be measured periodically.

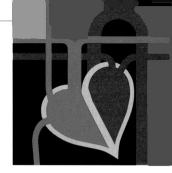

Common drugs for stroke *continued*

aspirin, a nonsteroidal anti-inflammatory

Important side effects	Negative drug interactions	Special warnings
Nausea, upset stomach, heartburn, appetite loss, bloody stool, continuous stomach pain, dizziness, hearing loss, ringing or buzzing in ears	**Do not combine with:** AZT *(zidovudine).* **Use caution with:** ACE inhibitors (Accupril, Capoten, Vasotec), adrenal corticosteroids, alcohol, anticoagulants *(dicumaron,* Miradon, *warfarin),* beta blockers (Inderal, Sectral, Tenormin), *methotrexate, nitroglycerin* tablets, *phenyl-butazone, probenecid, sulfinpyrazone.*	**Do not use if:** you have a GI bleeding disorder, a history of peptic ulcers, ulcer disease, or bleeding disorders, liver damage, or sever kidney failure. **Use caution if:** you have a history of asthma. Do not take aspirin for more than 10 consecutive days, or for more than 3 days if you have a fever. Do not use aspirin chewing gum for more than 2 days. Do not use aspirin before surgery. Take aspirin with food, milk, or water.

Tips for reducing your risk of stroke

- Have your blood pressure checked once a year.
- Don't smoke.
- Eat a well-balanced diet, but don't overeat.
- Know the warning signs of stroke and get immediate medical attention if you experience any of these: sudden weakness or numbness in the face, arm, or leg on one side of the body; sudden change in or loss of vision, loss of speech, or difficulty talking or understanding speech; sudden, severe headaches with no apparent cause; unexplained dizziness, unsteadiness, or sudden falls.

Urinary Tract

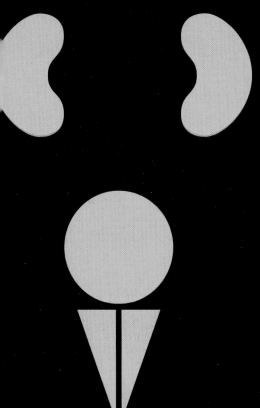

Our kidneys are necessary for life and are tied in closely with the bladder, ureters, urethra, and pelvic muscles. The entire system must be functioning efficiently for good health. An untreated case of incontinence can lead to bladder or urinary tract infections; these infections can progress to cause kidney disease.

he kidneys clean the blood by removing waste and extra fluids, regulate blood pressure, and balance body chemicals. These two organs are small—each about the size of a fist—but powerful, and when they're compromised due to disease or damage, the body suffers. First, waste and excess fluids build up inside the body, causing a host of unpleasant symptoms. Next, if left untreated, the kidneys may simply shut down, which could lead to death.

Just as the kidneys remove waste, they also eliminate drugs from the body. That's why it's critical for patients to inform their doctors if they have any kind of kidney disorder. In these cases, doctors may adjust drug dosages to avoid toxicity.

Drugs used to treat disorders of the kidneys and urinary tract range from antibiotics to diuretics. The following is a sampling.

> " The trouble with being a hypochondriac is that antibiotics have cured all the good diseases.
>
> CASKIE STINNET
> Out of the Red "

Impotence

Symptoms: Failure to get or maintain an erection.

Common drugs for impotence

Report any side effects to doctor if severe or persistent. Those in orange, report immediately.

Important side effects	Negative drug interactions	Special warnings
Viagra *(sildenafil)*, an erectile therapy agent		**$$$$**
Flushing, headache, nasal congestion, stomach discomfort, abnormal vision, (e.g., inability to distinquish blue and green), rash, indigestion, sensitivity to light, bladder pain, discolored urine, increased or painful urination, prolonged or painful erection	*Do not combine with:* Other erectile therapy agents, Glucotrol, Imdur *(isosorbide mononitrate)*, nitrates (Nitrostat, Transderm-Nitro). *Use caution with:* drugs that block or enhance the liver cytochrome system, *erythromycin*, nitrates, Nizoral *(ketoconazole)*, Norvasc *(amlopidine)*, other impotence medications, Posicor *(mibefradil)*, *rifampin*, Sporanox *(itraconazole)*, and Tagamet *(cimetidine)*.	*Do not use if:* you are over 65 years old or the drug was prescribed without a thorough medical history and exam. *Use caution if:* you have liver or kidney disease, cataracts or impaired vision, structural damage to the penis, stomach problems, retinal disease, have a history of heart disease, or are prone to heartburn.

Viagra Trivia

The prize for scoring a hole-in-one at a charity golf tour in Kuala Lumpur, Malaysia, will no longer be a year's supply of Viagra. Organizers of the **Catholic Doctors' Association** event say they had to pull the prize after receiving complaints that **they were promoting irresponsible use of the drug**.

They are not alone. Unscrupulous online pharmacies, in cahoots with unscrupulous cyber-doctors, have sold Viagra to a 16-year-old who charged the pills on his mother's credit card; a dead man, one who disclosed that he was taking a medication that could be fatal if taken with Viagra; and a cat, whose owner claimed on the application weighed **14 pounds, was six inches tall, and had been neutered**. $167 later, the pills arrived for the cat, who was named—what else'?—Iom.

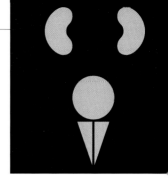

Incontinence

Incontinence—the term used to describe the involuntary loss of urine—comes in four different forms:

Our kidneys are

necessary for life.

An untreated case

of incontinence

can lead to bladder

or urinary tract

infections; these

infections can lead

further to kidney

disease.

- **Overflow incontinence** is somewhat self-explanatory. When the bladder fills to capacity and the kidneys continue to produce more urine, urine begins to dribble out. Sufferers are unable to eliminate urine adequately. This type of incontinence particularly affects older men with enlarged prostates. The enlarged prostate compresses the urethra, thus making the elimination of urine difficult.

- **Stress incontinence** is the sudden elimination of urine when the sufferer coughs, sneezes, laughs, or otherwise strains. It is more common in women because weakened pelvic muscles are unable to prevent voluntary urine elimination.

- **Total incontinence,** in which the bladder empties completely, is usually due to nerve or muscle damage, cancer, or other disorders. This type of incontinence usually requires corrective surgery.

- **Urge incontinence** usually occurs when the sufferer feels a sudden need to urinate, and the bladder muscle has a spasm, causing leakage. It is often caused by an infection, inflammation, prostate enlargement, or bladder control problems.

Common drugs for incontinence

Report any side effects to doctor if severe or persistent. Those in orange, report immediately.

Important side effects	Negative drug interactions	Special warnings
Detrol *(tolterodine),* an antispasmodic		$$$
Rash, blurred vision, increased light sensitivity, dry mouth	*Use caution with:* macrolide antibiotics (Biaxin, Ery-Tab, Zithromax), Monistat *(miconazole),* Nizoral *(ketoconazole),* and Sporanox *(itraconazole).*	*Do not use if:* you have urine retention, gastric retention, or uncontrolled glaucoma; are allergic to codeine or similar compounds or intoxicated by morphine-like drugs; or have

continued on next page

Common drugs for incontinence *continued*

Important side effects	Negative drug interactions	Special warnings
Detrol *continued*		
		taken an MAO inhibitor within the last 14 days.
		Use caution if: you are prone to constipation, have liver or kidney problems, a history of seizures or take medicine that makes seizures more likely, a history of alcoholism, epilepsy, thyroid gland problems, or will have surgery in the near future.
Ditropan *(oxybutynin chloride)*, antispasmodic $		
Ditropan XL *(oxybutynin chloride)*, antispasmodic $$$		
Constipation, decreased swelling, drowsiness, dry mouth, nose and throat, eye pain, rash, hives	*Do not combine with:* alcohol. *Use caution with:* antidepressants (Elavil, Nardil, Prozac), antihistamines (Claritin, Tavist, Zyrtec), antipsychotics (Clozaril, Haldol, Risperdal), anti-Parkinsonisms (Dopar, Sinemet, Symmetrel), Atrovent *(ipratropium)*, Norpace *(disopyramide)*, Orphenadrine, Procan SR *(procainamide)*, Quinate *(quinidine)*, Ritalin *(methylphenidate)*, Tegretol *(carbamazepine)*, and all sedatives.	*Do not use if:* you have untreated glaucoma, partial or complete blockage of the gastrointestinal tract, obstructed bowel, severe colitis, myasthenia gravis, or urinary tract infection. *Use caution if:* you have an ileostomy or colostomy, liver or kidney disease, or a nervous system disorder. Do not operate heavy machinery until you know how this medicine affects you. Avoid exposure to bright sunlight. Do not become overheated.

Liver or kidney disorders could cause adverse drug reactions

A common warning on both over-the-counter and prescription medications is that patients should use caution if they have a liver or kidney disorder. This warning points to a very serious problem posed by malfunctioning livers and kidneys. The liver breaks down some medications so the body can eliminate them, so when the liver is not functioning properly, dangerous levels of a medication could accumulate in the body and possibly cause a serious reaction in the patient.

Similarly, malfunctioning kidneys are unable to process drugs properly and prepare them for elimination through the urine. In either case, the patient runs the risk of retaining too much of a medication in the body and experiencing adverse reactions.

Kidney disorders include cancer, kidney disease, kidney infections, and kidney stones.

- **Symptoms of kidney cancer:** red or cloudy urine, dull pain in the abdomen, lower back, or side, a mass in the lower back, fatigue, low-grade fever, vomiting, and appetite and weight loss.
- **Symptoms of kidney disease:** frequent thirst and urge to urinate, passing small amounts of urine, swelling of hands and feet, puffy eyes, bad breath, fatigue, short-

ness of breath, appetite loss, increased blood pressure, and pale, dry, and itchy skin.

- **Symptoms of kidney infection:** pain in lower back, rising fever, frequent urge to urinate, cloudy or bloody urine, nausea, and vomiting.
- **Symptoms of kidney stones:** waves of severly sharp pain from side to groin, nausea, vomiting, sweating, and bloody urine.

If you have a liver or kidney disorder, your doctor may choose to prescribe a lower dose of some medications, and avoid other medications altogether. Be sure to discuss your options with your doctor before taking any kind of medication.

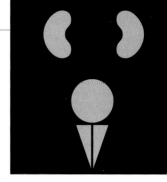

Prostate problems

The prostate is a walnut-sized gland that surrounds the male urethra. It produces a fluid that carries sperm. When enlarged, it obstructs the outward flow of urine. Two main types of prostate problems occur: enlargement of the prostate and prostatitis.

Symptoms of an enlarged prostate: difficulty urinating.

Symptoms of prostatitis: frequent, difficult, and painful urination, sudden fever and chills, pain in the lower back, blood in the urine, painful ejaculation, bloody semen, and sexual dysfunction.

Common drugs for prostate problems

Report any side effects to doctor if severe or persistent. Those in orange, *report immediately.*

Important side effects	Negative drug interactions	Special warnings
Cardura *(doxazosin)*, benign prostatic hyperplasia (BPH) therapy agent		$$
Flomax *(tamsulosin)*, benign prostatic hyperplasia (BPH) therapy agent		???
Hytrin *(terazosin)*, benign prostatic hyperplasia (BPH) therapy agent		$$$
Dizziness, headache, loss of strength or weakness, nasal congestion, peripheral swelling, drowsiness, diarrhea, back pain, stuffy or runny nose, nausea, irregular heartbeat, chest pain, prolonged or painful erection	*Do not combine with:* tobacco. *Use caution with:* Adalat CC, Calan *(verapamil)*, cold and allergy medications, Indocin *(indomethacin)*, nonsteroidal anti-inflammatories (Aleve, Daypro, Toradol), Procardia XL *(nifedipine)* and other blood pressure medications, Tagamet *(cimetidine)*, Valium *(diazepam)*, Vasotec *(enalapril)*, and Zantac *(ranitidine)*.	*Do not use if:* you have had a bad reactions to these drugs or Minipres *(prazosin)*. *Use caution if:* you have had lightheadedness upon standing while using other antihypertensive drugs, have impaired circulation to the brain, coronary artery disease, kidney problems, angina, a history of mental depression, stroke, high blood pressure, low white blood cells, or will have surgery in the near future. Use caution when operating heavy machinery.

Common drugs for prostate problems *continued*

Important side effects	Negative drug interactions	Special warnings

Eulexin *(flutamide)*, an antiandrogen, used to treat metastatic prostate cancer **$$$$$**

Important side effects	Negative drug interactions	Special warnings
Diarrhea, erectile dysfunction, loss of sexual desire, sudden sweating, feeling of warmth, blue lips, fingernails or palms, dark urine, dizziness, fainting, feeling of pressure in head, itching, appetite loss, nausea, vomiting, pain in right flank, shortness of breath, weak and rapid heartbeat, yellow skin or eyes	*Use caution with:* Coumadin *(warfarin).*	*Use caution if:* you have impaired liver function, high blood pressure, or a history of liver problems, anemia, low white blood cells, low blood platelets, or lupus erythematosus.

Proscar *(finasteride)*, a 5-alpha reductase inhibitor, used to treat symptomatic benign prostatic hyperplasia (BPH) and to decrease risk of urine retention in BPH **$$$$$**

Important side effects	Negative drug interactions	Special warnings
Impotence, decreased libido, rash		*Do not use if:* you are a woman. *Use caution if:* you have liver or kidney problems or if your sexual partner is pregnant. A prostate cancer exam is recommended before use of Proscar. If your sexual partner is pregnant, avoid exposing her to semen. Take Proscar on an empty stomach.

Pumpkin seed

Pygeum

Mild stomach irritation		

Saw Palmetto

Stomach irritation		

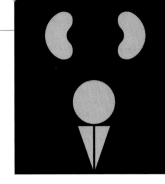

No more procrastinating

Men are notorious for avoiding the doctor's office. In fact, according to one estimate, men make 150 million fewer visits annually to doctors than women in the United States. Why are men so reluctant to see a doctor? There are any number of valid answers to this question: Men don't like to discuss their health, they tend to wait until a condition worsens before they seek treatment, they often don't want to follow doctor's orders, and they fear what their doctors might say.

It's easy to joke about men's fear of the doctor's office, but when it comes to prostate cancer, there's nothing funny to joke about. The media is full of information about breast cancer, but prostate cancer is actually more common. It's estimated that one in five American men will develop prostate cancer during their lifetimes, whereas one in eight American women are expected to develop breast cancer. Prostate cancer is the most common type of cancer among American men, and the second main cause of cancer deaths. (Lung cancer is the leading cause of cancer deaths among men.)

Urinary tract infection

Symptoms: a burning sensation when urinating, frequent urge to urinate, urine with a strong, foul odor, and, in the elderly, lethargy, incontinence, and mental confusion.

Common drugs for urinary tract infection

Report any side effects to doctor if severe or persistent. Those in orange, report immediately.

Important side effects	Negative drug interactions	Special warnings
Amoxicillin—see Sinusitis		
Ampicillin—see Sinusitis		
Azo Gantrisin *(sulfisoxazole)*, anti-infective		$
Bactrim DS *(sulfamethoxazole)*, anti-infective		$
Septra *(trimethoprim)*, anti-infective		$
Dizziness, diarrhea, headache, appetitie loss, nausea, vomiting, fatigue, itching, rash, aching joints and muscles, difficulty swallowing, pale or reddened skin, blistered or peeling skin, sore throat, fever, unusual bleeding or bruising, fatigue, yellow eyes or skin, pain in stomach or abdomen, bloody urine, increased or decreased urination, painful urination, unusual thirst, lower	*Use caution with:* Coumadin *(warfarin), methotrexate,* and oral antidiabetics (Amaryl, Glucophage, Glucotrol), and *phenytoin.*	***Do not use if:*** you are allergic to sulfonamide drugs. ***Use caution if:*** you have allergies, impaired liver or kidney function, a drug-induced blood cell or bone marrow disorder, a G6PD deficiency in your red blood cells, a history of porphyria, or will have pentothal anesthesia in the near future. Drink a lot of water while taking Azo-Gantrisin. May discolor your urine.

79

continued on next page

Common drugs for urinary tract infection *continued*

Important side effects	Negative drug interactions	Special warnings
Azo Gantrisin, Bactrim DS, Septra *continued*		
back pain, mood or mental changes, swelling in neck, increased sensitivity to sunlight		

Cipro *(ciprofloxacin),* fluoroquinolone antibiotics		$$$
Levaquin *(lomefloxacin),* fluoroquinolone antibiotics		$$$$
Floxin *(ofloxacin),* fluoroquinolone antibiotics		$$$$
Nausea, vomiting, diarrhea, abdominal discomfort, increased sensitivity to sunlight (skin burning, redness, blisters, rash, itching upon exposure to sunlight), seizures, mental confusion, hallucinations, agitation, nightmares, depression, shortness of breath, unusual swelling in face or extremities, loss of consciousness	*Do not combine with:* *theophylline.* *Use caution with:* antacids containing magnesium, aluminum or calcium, Benemid *(probenecid),* caffeine, calcium supplements, Carafate *(sucralfate),* Coumadin *(warfarin),* cyclosporine, Cytoxan *(cyclophosphamide),* Dilantin *(phenytoin),* glyburide, iron supplements, Lopressor *(metoprolol),* nonsteroidal anti-inflammatories (Aleve, Daypro, Toradol), oral antidiabetics (Amaryl, Glucotrol, Micronase), other quinolone antibiotics, products containing iron, and multivitamins containing zinc.	*Do not use if:* you have had an allergic reaction to a quinolone antibiotic, have a prolonged heartbeat interval, or have a central nervous system disorder or brain injury. *Use caution if:* you have a brain circulatory disorder, impaired liver or kidney function, a history of mental illness, or if you do heavy manual labor. Call your doctor if you experience a change in mental status. Drink a lot of water while taking these drugs.

Bearberry		
Nausea, vomiting	*Do not combine with:* citrus fruits, cranberries and blueberries.	Eat plenty of fruits and vegetables and drink fruit juices while taking Bearberry.

Cranberry		
		Cranberry will not cure an active infection, so antibiotics will be needed.

Parsley		
Skin irritation		*Do not use if:* you have water retention due to a heart or kidney condition, kidney inflammation or if you are allergic to others in this family like carrot, fennel, or celery.

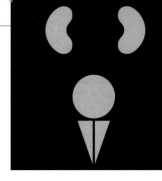

Common drugs for urinary tract infection *continued*		
Important side effects	**Negative drug interactions**	**Special warnings**
Dandelion		
Heartburn, gastric complaints		*Do not use if:* you have an obstruction of the bowels, bile duct, gallbladder, or ileus.

Does cranberry juice really work?

For years we've been told that drinking cranberry juice can prevent—and even help treat—urinary tract infections. Is that really true? The answer is, probably.

For years scientists have acknowledged a relationship between cranberry juice and the prevention and treatment of urinary tract infections. They once believed that the juice's ability to make urine more acid explained its healing powers,

but today, they are onto another explanation. Recent investigations have led researchers to speculate that cranberry juice prevents bacteria from sticking to the lining of the urinary tract, thus preventing them from multiplying and causing infection.

Whatever the magic of cranberry juice, it holds up in scientific studies. A study published in the **Journal of the American Medical Association** in 1994 demonstrated that women who drank cranberry juice every day for six months were half as likely

to develop a urinary tract infection as women who didn't drink the juice.

Experts advise that patients with urinary tract infections should never use cranberry juice as their only treatment. They should also consult a doctor for an antibiotic.

What about those cranberry pills sold in some health food stores and pharmacies? Sorry, there is no scientific evidence that they are effective in preventing and treating urinary tract infections.

When this signaling process goes askew, the effects are seen in a person's behavior and experienced in his emotions, perceptions, sensations, and ideas. Although there are numerous chemicals that perform vital functions within the brain, the three chemicals, or neurotransmitters, that seem most critical in maintaining mental balance are:

- **Serotonin,** which is related to anxiety, depression, and aggression.
- **Dopamine,** which affects reality perception and pleasurable experiences.
- **Norepinephrine,** which affects attention, concentration, and mood.

Whenever an imbalance appears evident through a person's disordered behavior and emotional state, medication centers on modifying the effects of these transmitters or readjusting the balance among these chemicals.

Here are some of the drugs most commonly used to treat mental health conditions.

Most of the nearly 2 million elderly Americans who suffer from severe depression are not treated.

OF THE **227,000 hip fractures** THAT OCCUR EACH YEAR (VIRTUALLY ALL IN OLDER ADULTS), ABOUT **32,000** ARE CAUSED BY THE USE OF MIND-AFFECTING DRUGS, ACCORDING TO A STUDY OF **1,000** OLDER ADULTS CITED IN *WORST PILLS, BEST PILLS.*

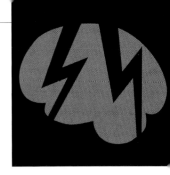

Anxiety disorder

Symptoms: All of us experience anxiety. Anxiety *disorder* is diagnosed when unrealistic worry and excessive fears, heart palpitations, breathlessness, muscle tension, insomnia, and irritability interfere with daily activities. Sufferers often have unrealistic fears that something bad will happen, such as a routine medical exam resulting in a cancer diagnosis.

STOP General Warnings

- Do not drink alcohol while taking antidepressants.
- Call your doctor immediately if you develop rash or hives with any of these drugs.
- Do not take monoamine oxidase inhibitor (MAOI) antidepressants, such as Nardil, until at least five weeks after your last dose of any selective serotonin re-uptake inhibitor (SSRIs), like Prozac, Zoloft, and Paxil.
- Do not stop taking any mind-affecting drug without informing your doctor. Many can cause serious reactions when withdrawn suddenly.

> The statistics on sanity are that one out of every four Americans is suffering from some form of mental illness. Think of your three best friends. If they're okay, then it's you.
>
> RITA MAE BROWN

Common drugs for anxiety

Report any side effects to doctor if severe or persistent. Those in orange, report immediately.

Important side effects	Negative drug interactions	Special warnings
BuSpar *(buspirone)*, an antianxiety drug		$$$$
Dizziness, lightheadedness, nausea, paradoxical increase in nervousness or exitability, restlessness, headache	*Use caution with:* antidepressants (Desyrel, Zoloft), Coumadin *(warfarin)*, Desyrel *(trazodone)*, macrolide antibiotics (Erytab, Biaxin, Zithromax), MAO inhibitors (Marplan, Nardil, Parnate), other drugs that affect the brain or nervous system.	*Do not take if:* you have taken an MAO inhibitor in the last 14 days. *Use caution if:* you have liver or kidney problems.

Common drugs for anxiety *continued*

Important side effects	Negative drug interactions	Special warnings

Xanax *(alprazolam)*, benzodiazepine tranquilizer $

Valium *(diazepam)*, benzodiazepine tranquilizer $

Ativan *(lorazepam)*, benzodiazepine tranquilizer $$

Important side effects	Negative drug interactions	Special warnings
Drowsiness, loss of coordination, unsteadiness, dizziness, lightheadedness, slurred speech, difficulty concentrating, outbursts of anger, behavioral problems, depression, hallucinations, low blood pressure causing faintness or confusion, memory impairment, muscle weakness, rash, itching, sore throat, fever, chills, sores or ulcers in mouth, unusual bleeding or bruising, fatigue, yellow eyes or skin	*Do not combine with:* alcohol, Biaxin *(clarithromycin)*, Nizoral *(ketoconazole)*, Sporanox and *(itraconazole)* Tagamet *(cimetidine)*. *Use caution with:* Antabuse *(disulfiram)*, anticonvulsants (Depakene, Dilantin, Tegretol), antidepressants (Nardil, Prozac, Zoloft), barbiturates (Amytal, Seconal, phenobarbital), Cardene *(nicardipine)*, Cardizem *(diltiazem)*, certain antibiotics, Cordarone *(amiodarone)*, cyclosporine, Darvon *(propoxyphene)*, ergotamine, grapefruit juice, *levodopa*, Luvox *(fluvoxamine)*, MAO inhibitors (Marplan, Nardil, Parnate), narcotics, *nifedipine*, other central nervous system depressants, other tranquilizers (BuSpar, Haldol, Valium), Paxil *(paroxetine)*, Prilosec *(omeprazole)*, Rifadin *(rifampin)*, Rifamate *(isoniazid)*, Serzone *(nefazodone)*, and Zoloft *(sertraline)*.	*Use caution if:* you are allergic to benzodiazepines; have liver or kidney problems; a history of palpitations, tachycardia, mental illness, alcoholism, or drug abuse; or have open-angle glaucoma, seizure disorder, or chronic lung disease. These can be addictive; do not stop use of them abruptly.

Kava Kava

	Do not combine with: alcohol, barbiturates (Butisol, Seconal, *phenobarbital*), or other mood-altering drugs (BuSpar, Prozac, Valium).	*Do not use if:* you have a depressive disorder. Do not use it for more than three months without consulting a doctor.

Valerian

Headache, insomnia, restlessness		*Do not use if:* you have a skin disorder, a severe infection, heart problems, or severe muscle tension.

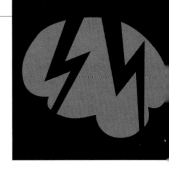

The ABCs on BDZs

Here's the scoop on benzodi-azepines (BDZs), the main class of drugs used to treat anxiety and insomnia, but only if you are under 65. (BDZs aren't recommended for those over 65.)

Benzodiazepines (BDZs) can be placed into two categories: tranquilizers for anxiety and sedatives for sleep disorders. The tranquilizers (Xanax, Ativan, Klonopin, Librium, Valium, Tranxene, Serax, Centrax) started appearing on the market in the early 1960s. Owing to a demand for sleep medications, new BDZs were developed to relieve insomnia. These include Halcion, Restoril, ProSom, Dalmane, and Doral.

The BDZ sleep aids, which are all highly addictive, treat different types of insomnia, depending on their duration of action. Short-acting sleep aids (such as Halcion) are active for four to six hours.

Intermediate sleep aids (Restoril, ProSom) take about two hours to absorb and are effective in treating middle insomnia. They last longer in the body, maintaining sleep for a longer period of time. Some of their effects can last into the following day.

Long-acting sleep aids (Dalmane, Doral) can last in the body for up to three to four days. In some cases, they still cause some drowsiness two or

three days after the initial dose. With regular use these sleep aids can build up in the body, especially in older people. For this reason these drugs are not recommended for those over age 60.

All BDZs—both tranquilizers and sedatives carry the same three warnings: (1) They will lose their effectiveness, a sign the body has developed tolerance; (2) They could lead to dependence; and (3) Abrupt discontinuation of the drugs can lead to withdrawal symptoms.

> There is nothing wrong with you that a little Prozac and a polo mallet won't cure.

WOODY ALLEN
Manhattan Murder Mystery

Major depression

Most of the nearly 2 million elderly Americans who suffer from severe depression are not treated, reports the **National Institute of Mental Health.**

Symptoms: Increased fatigue, suicidal thoughts, sadness, changes in appetite, sleep habits and sex drive, feelings of guilt and worthlessness, difficulty concentrating, and slowed thinking.

Common drugs for depression

Report any side effects to doctor if severe or persistent. Those in orange, *report immediately.*

Important side effects	Negative drug interactions	Special warnings
Amitriptyline, a tricyclic antidepressant and antimanic agent		$
Dizziness, lightheadedness, headache, dry mouth, unpleasant taste, increased sensitivity to light, weight gain, appetite increase, nausea, confusion, irregular heartbeat, hallucinations, seizures,	*Do not combine with:* alcohol. *Use caution with:* all other medications. Amitriptyline interacts with many other medications.	*Do not use if:* you are over 65, are taking or have taken an MAO inhibitor in the last 14 days, or have heart problems. *Use caution if:* you have liver, kidney or blood cell disorders; a history of diabetes, epilepsy,

continued on next page

Common drugs for depression *continued*

Important side effects	Negative drug interactions	Special warnings

Amitriptyline *continued*

fatigue, drowsiness, blurred or altered vision, breathing difficulty, constipation, impaired concentration, difficult urination, fever, restlessess, loss of coordination or balance, difficulty swallowing or speaking, dilated pupils, eye pain, fainting, trembling, shaking, weakness, stiffness in extremities, shuffling gait		glaucoma, heart disease, prostate gland enlargement, overactive thyroid function, schizophrenia, prostate or sexual problems, or intestinal block; or will have surgery or shock therapy in the near future.

Celexa *(citalopram hydrobromide)*, a selective serotonin reuptake inhibitor $$$$

Abdominal pain, agitation, anxiety, chest pain, diarrhea, drowsiness, dry mouth, ejaculation disorders, fainting, fatigue, heartbeat changes, indigestion, insomnia, lightheadedness, loss of appetite, nausea, numbness, painful menstruation, respiratory tract infection, sinus or nasal inflammation, sweating, tingling, tremor, vomiting	*Do not combine with:* alcohol and MAO inhibitors (Marplan, Nardil, Parnate). *Use caution with:* Coumadin *(warfarin)*, Diflucan *(fluconazole)*, erthromycin, lithium, Lopressor *(metoprolol)*, Nizoral *(ketoconazole)*, other antidepressants (Elavil, Nardil, Prozac), Prilosec *(omeprazole)*, Sporanox *(itraconazole)*, Tagamet *(cimetidine)*, and Tegretol *(carbamazepine)*.	*Use caution if:* you have or have a history of heart disease, high blood pressure, mania, seizures, liver disease, liver or kidney problems, or are over 60 years old. Do not drive or operate heavy machinery until you know how you react to this drug.

Desyrel *(trazodone)*, an antidepressant $

Drowsiness, dry mouth, dizziness, lightheadedness, unpleasant taste in mouth, nausea, vomiting, headache, muscle twitching, confusion	*Do not combine with:* alcohol. *Use caution with:* antihypertensive drugs (Cardura, Catapres, Hytrin), barbiturates (Amytal, Seconal, *phenobarbital*), central nervous system depressants, Coumadin *(warfarin)*, Dilantin *(phenytoin)*, high blood pressure medications, Lanoxin *(digoxin)*, MAO inhibitors (Marplan, Nardil, Parnate), other antidepressants (Elavil, Nardil, Prozac), and Thorazine *(chlorpromazine)*.	*Do not use if:* you are recovering from a recent heart attack or have taken an MAO inhibitor in the last 14 days. *Use caution if:* you have liver or kidney problems; have a history of alcoholism, epilepsy, or heart disease; or will have surgery in the near future.

Effexor *(venlafaxine)*, a bicyclic antidepressant $$$

Fatigue, dizziness, drowsiness, anxiety, dry mouth, changed sense of taste, appetite loss, nausea, vomiting, chills, diarrhea, constipation, prickly skin sensation, heartburn,	*Do not combine with:* alcohol, Eldepryl *(selegiline)*, and MAO inhibitors (Marplan, Nardil, Parnate).	*Use caution if:* you have a history of high blood pressure, abnormally increased lipids, seizures, mania, or hypomania; have liver or kidney problems or trouble sleeping;

continued on next page

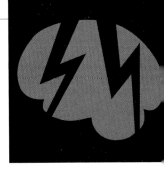

Common drugs for depression *continued*

Important side effects	Negative drug interactions	Special warnings

Effexor *continued*

increased sweating, runny nose, stomach gas or pain, insomnia, unusual dreams, weight loss, headache, changes in vision, decreased sexual ability or desire, difficulty urinating, itching, rash, chest pain, heartbeat irregularities, mood or mental changes, drowsiness, fatigue	*Use caution with:* other drugs that affect the central nervous system, including narcotics, sleep aids, tranquilizers, antipsychotics, and other antidepressants, and Tagamet (*cimetidine*).	or have had a recent heart attack.

Paxil *(paroxetine),* a selective serotonin reuptake inhibitor $$$$

Nausea, drowsiness, headache, dry mouth, asthenia, constipation, insomnia, dizziness, diarrhea, trembling, sexual dysfunction , anorexia, sedation, nervousness and anxiety, fatigue, loss of initiative, vomiting, constipation, difficulty urinating, muscle pain or fatigue, lightheadedness, fainting, rash, agitation, irritability, dilated pupils, dry mouth, rapid heartbeat	*Do not combine with:* alcohol *Use caution with:* antidepressants (Elavil, Nardil, Prozac), Coumadin *(warfarin),* Dilantin *(phenytoin),* diuretics, Imitrex *(sumatriptan),* Kemadrin *(procyclidine),* Lanoxin *(digoxin),* Lithonate *(lithium),* Mellaril *(thioridazine),* phenobarbital, propanolol, Quinaglute *(quinidine),* Rythmol *(propafenone),* Tagamet *(cimetidine),* Tambocor *(flecainide), tryptophan,* and Valium *(diazepam).*	*Do not take if:* you have taken an MAO inhibitor in the last 14 days. *Use caution if:* you have liver or kidney problems or a history of mania or seizures.

Prozac *(fluoxetine),* a selective serotonin reuptake inhibitor $$$$

Headache, nausea, insomnia , drowsiness, nervousness and anxiety, diarrhea and asthenia, anorexia, dizziness, dry mouth and tremor, upper respiratory infection, dyspepsia, influenza, excessive sweating, decreased appetite, decreased initiative, agitation, shaking, difficulty breathing, rash, hives, itching, joint or muscle pain, chills, fever	*Do not combine with:* alcohol or MAO inhibitors (Marplan, Nardil, Parnate). *Use caution with:* Buspar *(buspirone),* Clozaril *(clozapine),* Coumadin *(warfarin),* Crystodigin *(digitoxin),* Dilantin *(phenytoin),* drugs that impair brain function, Eskalith *(lithium),* Haldol *(haloperidol),* Orap *(pimozide),* other antidepressants (Elavil, Nardil, Prozac), Tambocor *(flecainide),* Tegretol *(carbamazepine), tryptophan,* Valium *(diazepam),* Velban *(vinblastine),* and Xanax *(alprazolam).*	*Do not use if:* you have taken an MAO inhibitor in the past 14 days. Do not combine with shock treatment. *Use caution if:* you have liver or kidney problems, Parkinson's disease, a seizure disorder, or a history of psychosis. Tell your doctor if you have an unexplained weight loss.

Common drugs for depression *continued*

Important side effects	Negative drug interactions	Special warnings

Serzone *(nefazodone)*, an antidepressant $$$$

Drowsiness, dizziness, agitation, dry mouth, confusion, constipation, diarrhea, unusual dreams, heartburn, fever, chills, insomnia, loss of memory, headache, flushing, nausea, vomiting, increased appetite, changes in vision, unsteadiness, clumsiness, rash, lightheadedness, ringing in ears

Do not combine with: Mevacor *(lovastatin)* and Zocor *(simvastatin)*

Use caution with: alcohol, Celexa *(citoprolam)*, Lanoxin *(digoxin)*, MAO inhibitors (Marplan, Nardil, Parnate), and other antidepressants.

Do not use if: you have taken an MAO inhibitor in the last 14 days.

Use caution if: you have liver or kidney problems, a history of seizure disorder, or heart disease.

Wellbutrin *(bupropion)*, an antidepressant $$

Nausea, vomiting, constipation, unusual weight loss, dry mouth, appetite loss, dizziness, increased sweating, trembling, shaking, hallucinations, irregular heartbeat, confusion, rash, insomnia, headache, excitement, agitation, seizures

Do not combine with: alcohol.

Use caution with: Cytoxan *(cyclophosphamide)*, Dilantin *(phenytoin)*, Larodopa *(levodopa)*, major tranquilizers (Mellaril, Serentil, Thorazine), MAO inhibitors (Marplan, Nardil, Parnate), Norgesic *(orphenadrine)*, other antidepressants (Elavil, Nardil, Prozac), *phenobarbital*, steroid medications, Tagamet *(cimetidine)*, Tegretol *(carbamazepine)*, and Theo-Dur *(theophylline)*.

Do not use if: you have liver or kidney problems, a seizure disorder, or a history of anorexia or bulimia, or have taken an MAO inhibitor in the last 14 days.

Use caution if: you have had a bad reaction to an antidepressant drug; have a history of mental illness, head injury, brain tumor, alcoholism, or drug abuse; have heart, liver, or kidney problems.

Age-related liver or kidney function decline may require dose decreases.

Zoloft *(sertraline)*, a selective serotonin reuptake inhibitor $$$$

Nausea, headache, insomnia and dry mouth, diarrhea, drowsiness, dizziness, tremor and fatigue, increased sweating and constipation, agitation and dyspepsia, sexual dysfunction, appetite decrease, weight loss, stomach cramps, abdominal pain, gas, loss of initiative, rash, hives, itching, unusually fast speech, fever, agitation

Do not combine with: alcohol, Eldepryl *(selegiline)*, MAO inhibitors (Marplan, Nardil, Parnate), and Meridia *(sibutramine)*.

Use caution with: Coumadin *(warfarin)*, diazepam, Lithonate *(lithium)*, Orinase *(tolbutamide)*, other antidepressants (Elavil, Nardil, Prozac), other serotonin-boosting drugs, including Paxil *(paroxetine)* and Prozac *(fluoxetine)*, over-the-counter medications, Rythmol *(propafenone)*, Tagamet *(cimetidine)*, and Tambocor *(flecainide)*.

Do not use if: you have taken an MAO inhibitor in the last 14 days. Do not combine with shock treatment.

Use caution if: you have had a bad reaction to an antidepressant drug; have liver or kidney problems, Parkinson's disease, or a seizure disorder; or have had a recent heart attack.

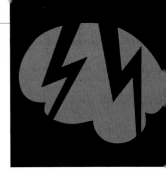

Common drugs for depression *continued*		
Important side effects	**Negative drug interactions**	**Special warnings**
s-adenosyl-methionine/SAMe		
Upset stomach nausea, vomiting		SAMe may trigger manic episodes in people with bipolar disorder.
St. John's wort		
Sensitivity to sunlight, bloating, constipation	***Do not combine with:*** MAO inhibitors (Marplan, Nardil, Parnate) and aged, pickled, and fermented food and beverages. Little is known as to how St. John's wort may interact with other medications.	Minimize exposure to the sun.

St. John's Wort: The Natural Prozac?

Prozac, Zoloft, and Paxil are the most prescribed antidepressants in the United States, and the reason is quite clear. These drugs, known as selective serotonin reuptake inhibitors (SSRIs), work by making sure the brain processes plenty of serotonin, a critical neurotransmitter. Serotonin helps regulate mood and behavior, and without enough of the chemical, we can become depressed, irritable, violent, and overindulgent with food, alcohol, or drugs. These medications affect the amount of serotonin in the space between nerve cells by preventing the recycling of this neurotransmitter.

St. John's wort is also considered an SSRI, giving itself the nickname of **the natural Prozac.** Some studies suggest that St. John's wort is also a monoamine oxidase inhibitor (MAOI). Monoamine oxidase is an enzyme that breaks down serotonin, so an MAOI attacks the monoamine oxidase before it has a chance to attack the serotonin.

St. John's wort has been used medicinally for more than 2,000 years and was named after **John the Baptist**, near whose birthday (June 24) the plant's golden flowers usually appear. (**Wort** is the Middle English word for **plant.**)

The plant grows wild around the world and is often considered a weed. Beware of harvesting your own St. John's wort, though. Efforts to eradicate it with herbicides have failed; the weed just won't succumb to poison. So any plants you find may be coated with a toxic herbicide.

Sleep disorders

Sleep disorders include insomnia, excessive daytime sleepiness, disorders in biological rhythms, nighttime agitation or confusion, and sleep apnea (episodes of interrupted breathing during sleep).

🛑 General Warnings

- Sleeping pills are not for chronic sleeping problems. They should be used only when needed and should not be used continuously for more than two weeks.
- Sleeping pills are especially problematic for those over 65.
- Do not drink alcohol while taking sleeping pills.
- Remember sleeping pills only help you fall asleep, not stay asleep.

THE NATIONAL INSTITUTE OF HEALTH ESTIMATES THAT SLEEP DISTURBANCES AFFECT **50%** OF ADULTS OVER AGE **65** LIVING AT HOME AND **66%** OF THOSE LIVING IN LONG-TERM-CARE FACILITIES.

Common drugs for sleep disorders

Report any side effects to doctor if severe or persistent. Those in orange, report immediately.

Important side effects	Negative drug interactions	Special warnings
Ambien *(zolpidem)*, a sleep-inducing drug		**$$$**
Daytime drowsiness, diarrhea, general pain or discomfort, memory problems, nausea, unusual dreams, vomiting, hallucinations, abnormal thoughts or behavior, confusion or disorientation, unsteadiness, dizziness, lightheadedness, unusual nervousness, agitation, difficulty breathing	*Do not combine with:* alcohol. *Use caution with:* other drugs that depress the central nervous system, including Valium, Percocet and Benadryl, Thorazine *(chlorpromazine)*, and Tofranil *(imipramine)*.	*Use caution if:* you have a history of alcoholism, drug abuse, mental disorders or if you have liver, kidney or lung problems. Take Ambien just before bedtime on an empty stomach. Withdrawal symptoms can occur upon stopping Ambien. You may be at increased risk for falls in the morning.
Dalmane *(flurazepam)*, benzodiazepine sleep-inducing drug		**$**
Doral *(quazepam)*, benzodiazepine sleep-inducing drug		**$**
Halcion *(triazolam)*, benzodiazepine sleep-inducing drug		**$**

continued on next page

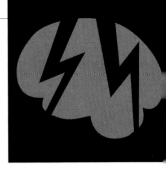

Common drugs for sleep disorders *continued*

Important side effects	Negative drug interactions	Special warnings

ProSom *(estazolam)*, benzodiazepine sleep-inducing drug $

Restoril *(temazepam)*, benzodiazepine sleep-inducing drug $

Important side effects	Negative drug interactions	Special warnings
Daytime drowsiness, dizziness, lightheadedness, loss of coordination, headaches, slurred speech, nausea, nervousness, sleepiness, weakness, difficulty concentrating, anger outbursts, behavioral problems, common cold, decreased mobility, depression, convulsions, hallucinations, hangover, low blood pressure, faintness, confusion, memory impairment, muscle weakness, rash, itching, sore throat, fever, chills, sores or ulcers in throat or mouth, unusual bruising or bleeding, unusual thoughts, fatigue, yellow eyes or skin	*Do not combine with:* alcohol or grapefruit juice. *Use caution with:* anticonvulsants (Depakene, Dilantin, Tegretol), antidepressants (Elavil, Nardil, Prozac), antihistamines (Benadryl, Claritin, Tavist), barbiturates (Amytal, Seconal, *phenobarbital*), Cordarone *(amiodarone)*, MAO inhibitors (Marplan, Nardil, Parnate), major tranquilizers (Mellaril, Serentil, Thorazine), mood-altering medications, narcotics, Nizoral *(ketoconazole)*, other central nervous system depressants, sedatives, Sporanox *(itraconazole)*, and tranquilizers. Halcion interacts with many other medications. Consult your doctor before combining this drug with any other.	*Do not use if:* you have had an allergic reaction to a Valium-type medication or if you have depression. Do not take if you have sleep apnea. *Use caution if:* you have depression; have liver, kidney, or lung problems; are over 65 or physically run-down; or have ever abused drugs or alcohol. Do not operate heavy machinery or do anything that requires full alertness after taking these medications. Do not stop use of these medications abruptly. Over time, these drugs may lose effectiveness, and/or cause dependence. Do not use these drugs on overnight flights of less than eight hours.

Bayer PM Extra Strength *(diphenhydramine)*

Excedrin PM *(diphenhydramine)*

Sominex Maximum Strength *(diphenhydramine)*

Tylenol PM Extra Strength *(diphenhydramine)*

Unisom Pain Relief *(diphenhydramine)*

Important side effects	Negative drug interactions	Special warnings
Restlessness, nervousness, sleeplessness, drowsiness, sedation, excitability, dizziness, poor coordination, upset stomach, confusion	*Use caution with:* barbiturates (Butisol, Seconal, *phenobarbital*, other sleep aids (Ambien, ProSom, Doral).	*Use caution if:* you have glaucoma, heart problems, or an enlarged prostate. Call your doctor if your insomnia lasts more than two weeks.

Bugleweed

Important side effects	Negative drug interactions	Special warnings
	Do not use with: thyroid preparations.	*Do not use if:* you have thyroid problems or plan to have diagnostic tests that require radioactive isotopes.

Halcion hassles

More than 11 other countries, including Britain and France have banned Halcion for its inclination to cause extreme sedation, violent and irrational behavior, suicidal thoughts, rebound insomnia and dependence. The FDA has regularly amended instructions to further limit the dosages and length of treatment, but a majority of physicians continue to prescribe it for longer periods than recommended (see Chapter 1). All hypnotics are recommended for short-term use, yet physicians regularly prescribe all BDZs for longer periods.

Common drugs for sleep disorders *continued*		
Important side effects	**Negative drug interactions**	**Special warnings**
Hops		
Lavender		
Passionflower		
Melatonin		
Headache, rash, upset stomach	*Use caution with:* beta blockers (Inderal, Sectral, Tenormin), Motrin *(ibuprofen)*, mood-altering drugs (BuSpar, Prozac, Valium), and steroid medications (Azmacort, Flonase, Ultravate).	*Do not use if:* you have AIDS, any autoimmune disease (like rheumatoid arthritis), a condition affecting the lymphatic system, depression, diabetes, epilepsy, heart disease, leukemia, multiple sclerosis, osteoarthritis, or serious allergies.
Valerian		
Headache restlessness, sleeplessness, excessive dilation of the pupils, disorders of cardiac function		

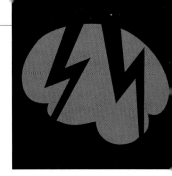

All in a night's sleep

A new study shows that consistently being deprived of sleep can increase the severity of age-related chronic disorders, including diabetes, obesity and high-blood pressure. The study at the **University of Chicago Medical School** in Chicago, Ill., of 11 men ages 18 to 27 found that after being deprived of sleep, the men experienced a rapid deterioration of bodily functions. They metabolized glucose less effectively, which suggests the possible development of diabetes. Levels of cortisol—a stress hormone that helps regulate blood sugar concentrations—were also higher than after periods of sustained sleep. Raised cortisol levels have been implicated in the memory impairments and age-related insulin resistance. Researcher **Eve Van Cauter**, who led the study, concluded that chronic sleep deprivation may have long-term harmful effects on the body.

23 million Americans. Acetominophen is often recommended as a first line treatment for osteoarthritis because of its safety. Traditional arthritis treatments—aspirin and ibuprofen—relieve pain, but plague patients with stomach upset and gastrointestinal bleeding. They are beginning to lose ground to Cox-2 inhibitors, a new class of drugs that relieve pain as well as aspirin and ibuprofen without the negative side effects.

Muscular discomfort caused by a sprain, a strain or another physical injury is often treated with an analgesic or NSAID (non-steroidal anti-inflammatory drug). A muscle relaxant may be prescribed when spasm is a significant factor.

Many people use the mnemonic RICES to approach acute musculoskeletal injury:

R Rest the affected area

I Ice the area for 20 minutes every hour for the first day. In a pinch, a bag of frozen peas makes a great ice bag (don't eat them afterward, though!)

C Compression by wrapping the area to prevent swelling

E Elevation of the affected limb will also decrease swelling

S Splinting can be used to prevent further injury, but just for the first day. Excessive splinting can cause muscles to lose their tone.

Read on for detailed information about medications used for musculoskeletal disorders.

> Musculoskeletal disorders, by some estimates, are responsible for the majority of lost work time among American workers.

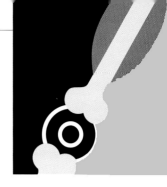

Arthritis

Osteoarthritis, also called degenerative joint disease, is an inflammation of the joint. It is generally caused by joint degeneration. Pain relievers can be used for osteoarthritis, but anti-inflammatory agents are not particularly useful even though they are commonly tried.

Symptoms of osteoarthritis: stiffness, joint pain, soft tissue swelling, and restricted mobility. Rheumatoid arthritis, also called rheumatism, is a chronic inflammatory condition that usually affects the joints. Anti-inflammatory agents do help combat this type of arthritis.

Symptoms of rheumatoid arthritis: fatigue, fever, weakness, joint swelling and morning stiffness, and joint pain.

STOP **General Warnings**

- **Report any signs of infection.**
- **Depression may be a risk factor for osteoporosis. If you have depression, it is wise to be checked for osteoporosis.**
- **Calcium supplements and Vitamin D may need to be added to your diet if you have osteoporosis.**

Common drugs for arthritis

Report any side effects to doctor if severe or persistent. Those in orange, *report immediately.*

Important side effects	Negative drug interactions	Special warnings
Celebrex *(celecoxib),* cox-2 inhibitors		$$$$
Vioxx *(rofecoxib),* cox-2 inhibitors		$$$$
Stomach pain, black and tarry stools, nausea, vomiting, fatigue, appetite loss, yellow skin or eyes, dark urine, rash, swelling, chest congestion, coughing, fever, sneezing, sore	*Do not use:* lithium *Use caution with:* ACE inhibitors (Accupril, Capoten, Prinivil), alcohol, aspirin and other salicylates, Coumadin	*Do not use if:* you have had an allergic reaction to a sulfa drug or aspirin or other nonsteroidal anti-inflammatories.

continued on next page

Common drugs for arthritis *continued*

Important side effects	Negative drug interactions	Special warnings

Celebrex, Vioxx *continued*

throat, anaphylaxis (which includes irregular breathing, fainting, changes in skin color, fast heartbeat, hive-like swelling, and swollen eyes), headache, indigestion, upper respiratory infection, diarrhea, sinus inflammation, back pain, diarrhea, dizziness, headache, heartburn, loss of energy, runny or stuffy nose	*(warfarin), fluconazole, furosemide, ketorolac, rifampin,* and tobacco.	*Use caution if:* you have allergies, or if you have had ulcers or stomach bleeding, or if you have alcohol abuse, bleeding or stomach problems, anemia, asthma, dehydration, kidney problems, high blood pressure, heart, liver or kidney disease, heart failure, or if you retain fluids.

Naproxen, nonsteroidal anti-inflammatory drug (NSAID) $

Daypro *(oxaprozin)*, nonsteroidal anti-inflammatory drug (NSAID) $$$$

Nausea, vomiting, heartburn, diarrhea, constipation, headache, dizziness, sleepiness, shortness of breath, wheezing, swelling of legs, chest pain, peptic ulcer disease with vomiting of blood, black and tarry stools, decreasing kidney function	*Do not combine with:* alcohol, antacids, aspirin, *methotrexate,* Coumadin *(warfarin).* *Use caution with:* ACE inhibitors (Accupril, Capoten, Vasotec), Benemid *(probenecid),* beta blockers (Inderal, Sectral, Tenormin), digitalis preparations, *digoxin,* Dilantin *(phenytoin),* diuretics (Bumex, Diuril, Diamox), Lasix *(furosemide),* Lithonate *(lithium), naproxen sodium,* oral antidiabetics (Amaryl, Glucotrol, Micronase).	*Do not use if:* you have developed asthma or nasal polyps after taking aspirin or if you have a bleeding, blood cell or kidney disorder. *Use caution if:* you are allergic to aspirin or aspirin substitutes; have active peptic ulcer disease, heart failure, impaired liver or kidney function, high blood pressure; or have a history of peptic ulcer disease, bleeding disorder or heart failure. Report signs of infection.

Prednisone, steroid $

Appetite increase, indigestion, nervousness, insomnia, increased infections, increased blood pressure, slowed healing of wounds, weight gain, easy bruising, fluid retention, vision problems, frequent urination, increased thirst, rectal bleeding, blistering skin, confusion, hallucinations, paranoia, euphoria, depression, mood swings, redness or swelling at injection site	*Use caution with:* anticonvulsants (Dilantin, Neurontin, Tegretol), antidiabetics (Glucophage, *insulin,* Glucotrol), aspirin, diuretics (Bumex, Diuril, Diamox), *estrogen,* oral contraceptives (Loestrin, Nordette, Ortho Cyclen), *phenobarbital,* Rifadin *(rifampin),* and Sandimmune *(cyclosporine).*	*Do not use if:* you have peptic ulcer disease, a herpes simplex virus eye infection, tuberculosis, or a fungal infection. *Use caution if:* you have had a bad reaction to any cortisone-like drug or have been exposed to a viral infection; have diabetes, kidney failure, glaucoma, high blood pressure, deficient thyroid function, myasthenia gravis, osteoporosis, or diverticulitis; a history of depression, peptic ulcer disease, thrombophlebitis, or tuberculosis; or will have surgery in the near future. Carry a card stating that you are taking prednisone. Avoid prolonged use of this drug. Do not stop taking this drug abruptly.

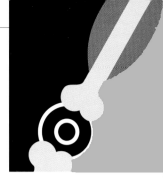

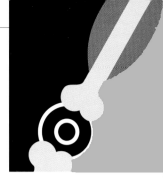

Common drugs for arthritis _continued_		
Important side effects	**Negative drug interactions**	**Special warnings**
Relafen _(nabumetone),_ a nonsteroidal anti-inflammatory drug (NSAID) $$$		
Nausea, vomiting, heartburn, diarrhea, constipation, headache, dizziness, sleepiness, shortness of breath, wheezing, swelling of legs, chest pain, peptic ulcer disease with vomiting of blood, black and tarry stools, decreased kidney function	_Do not combine with:_ alcohol, antacids, aspirin, methotrexate, Coumadin _(warfarin)._ _Use caution with:_ ACE inhibitors (Accupril, Capoten, Vasotec), Benemid _(probenecid),_ beta blockers (Inderal, Sectral, Tenormin), digitalis preparations, _digoxin,_ Dilantin _(phenytoin),_ diuretics (Bumex, Diuril, Diamox), Lasix _(furosemide),_ Lithonate _(lithium), naproxen sodium,_ oral antidiabetics (Amaryl, Glucotrol, Micronase).	_Do not use if:_ you have developed asthma or nasal polyps after taking aspirin; have active peptic ulcer disease, gastrointestinal ulcers or bleeding, liver disease, kidney bleeding, blood cell disorders, or porphyria; or have a history of rectal bleeding or proctitis. _Use caution if:_ you are allergic to aspirin or aspirin substitutes; have high blood pressure, liver or kidney problems; or have a history of peptic ulcer disease, Crohn's disease, ulcerative colitis, bleeding disorder, epilepsy, Parkinson's disease, mental illness, or heart failure.
Advil		
Arthritis Foundation Ibuprofen		
Bayer Select Ibuprofen Pain Relief		
Motrin _(ibuprofen)_		
Aleve _(naproxen sodium)_		
Constipation, indigestion, heartburn, nausea, diarrhea, stomach irritation, drowsiness	_Do not combine with:_ alcohol, antacids, aspirin, _methotrexate,_ Coumadin _(warfarin)._ _Use caution with:_ ACE inhibitors (Accupril, Capoten, Vasotec), Benemid _(probenecid),_ beta blockers (Inderal, Sectral, Tenormin), digitalis preparations, _digoxin,_ Dilantin _(phenytoin),_ diuretics (Bumex, Diuril, Diamox), Lasix _(furosemide),_ Lithonate _(lithium), naproxen sodium,_ oral antidiabetics (Amaryl, Glucotrol, Micronase).	_Use caution if:_ you have heart failure, high blood pressure, kidney damage, bleeding disorders, peptic ulcer disease, and diabetes. Do not take naproxen sodium for more than 10 days in a row.

Common drugs for arthritis *continued*

Important side effects	Negative drug interactions	Special warnings
Arthritis Foundation Aspirin Free		
Bayer Select Aspirin Free		
Excedrin		
Tylenol *(acetaminophen)*		
Lightheadedness	***Do not combine with:*** alcohol. ***Use caution with:*** barbiturates (Butisol, *phenobarbital*, Seconal), Coumadin *(warfarin)*, Dilantin *(phenytoin)*, INH *(isoniazid)*, Rifaden *(rifampin)*, sulfinpyrazone, and Tegretol *(carbamazepine)*.	***Use caution if:*** you have kidney or liver disease or an infection of the liver. Do not take acetaminophen for more than 10 days in a row.
⚠ *aspirin*—see stroke		
MSM *(methylsulfonylmethane)*		
Nausea, diarrhea, headache		
Boswellia		
Diarrhea, nausea, skin rash		
Cayenne		
Diarrhea, cramps, blisters		Do not overdose or use for an extended period of time.
Chondroitin		
	Use caution with: anticoagulants, such as Coumadin *(warfarin)*.	***Use caution if:*** you have a blood clotting disorder.

More than 2,000 years ago, aspirin was used to relieve pain. Today, it is not only used to ease pain, but also to reduce the risk of heart attack, to reduce the risk of blood clotting in heart attack survivors, and to prevent stroke. It is a fascinating drug with a long history.

The Greek physician Hippocrates prescribed the bark and leaves of the willow tree to relieve pain and fever. The willow tree is rich in a substance called salicin.

Willow leaves were described in writings by Romans Pliny the Elder and Galen, a doctor.

Felix Hoffman, a chemist at Bayer in Germany, chemically synthesized a stable form of ASA powder that relieved his father's rheumatism. The compound later became the active ingredient in aspirin. Aspirin's name is made up of "a," from acetyl, "spir," from the spirea plant (which yields salicin), and "in," a common suffix for medications.

200 BC	100 BC	100 AD	200	600	1000	1400	1800	1825	1850

Willow leaves were mentioned in writings of the Greek surgeon Dioscorides.

A German chemist experimented with salicin and created salicyclic acid (SA).

Bayer distributed aspirin powder to physicians to give to their patients. Aspirin soon became the number one drug worldwide.

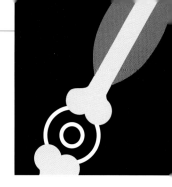

Common drugs for arthritis *continued*		
Important side effects	**Negative drug interactions**	**Special warnings**
Glucosamine		
Diarrhea, heartburn, indigestion, nausea		
Guaiac		
Diarrhea, gastroenteritis, skin rash		
White willow		
Stomach discomfort	*Use caution with:* salicylates and other nonsteroidal anti-inflammatories.	*Do not use if:* you are sensitive to aspirin.

Aspirin's here, it's there, it's everywhere: an aspirin timeline

Americans consume an estimated 80 billion aspirin tablets a year. That's about 307 per person per year. The Physicians' Desk Reference lists more than 50 over-the-counter drugs that list aspirin as the active ingredient. And new uses for the drug have been uncovered for most of its 100-year existence. Just read from the 2,700 articles on aspirin listed on the **National Library of Medicine's** computer catalog—and those include only articles in English that have been published in the last five years. The latest uses being studied: prevention of colon cancer, delay of progression of Alzheimer's, arrest of periodontal disease, prevention of cataracts, and control of preeclampsia and high blood pressure that occurs in some pregnancies.

Bayer introduced the first aspirin in water-soluble tablets. This was the first medication sold in that form, and it cut costs in half.

Dr. Lawrence Craven, a California general practitioner, noticed that the 400 men to whom he had prescribed aspirin had not suffered any heart attacks. He began to recommend that all his patients and colleagues take an aspirin a day to reduce the risk of heart attack.

The British pharmacologist John R. Vane was awarded the Nobel Prize for Medicine for discovering aspirin's basic mechanism of action. He noted that the action of acetylsalicylic acid is due to the inhibition of prostaglandin synthesis.

The FDA signaled its intent to broaden the use of aspirin for the prevention of strokes in women after a TIA, after a minor stroke in both men and women, in certain groups at high risk for heart attack and stroke, and in dosages lower than previously recommended.

1900   1925   1950   1975   2000

Aspirin became available without a prescription.

The Food and Drug Administration (FDA) approved the use of aspirin to reduce the risk of stroke after transient "ischemic attack" (TIA) in men.

The FDA approved the use of aspirin in preventing heart attacks in patients who have had a heart attack or unstable angina.

In 1996, the FDA proposed new labeling for the use of aspirin during a suspected heart attack.

Got gout?

Gout has been a recognized medical condition since at least as far back as **Hippocrates'** time. It's known as **the disease of kings and the king of diseases**, probably because it can be aggravated by rich foods and alcohol, is associated with obesity, and occurs mainly in men.

Despite its long history and aristocratic associations, gout is widely misunderstood. It's considered a form of arthritis, and can even be mistaken for certain other kinds of arthritis, but it requires a specific treatment plan for maximum relief.

Colchicine has been the treatment of choice among gout sufferers since the nineteenth century, but some patients don't appreciate the drug's common

side effects: nausea, vomiting, and diarrhea. For those who are dissatisfied with colchicine, there are always the non-steroidal anti-inflammatory (NSAIDs). They don't cause the unsavory side effects of colchicine, and are tolerated by most patients, if used on a short-term basis. Doctors warn, however, that aspirin products should be avoided in patients suffering acute gout attacks.

Gout

Symptoms: fever, chills, and excruciating pain usually in a single joint, sometimes low grade fever.

Common drugs for gout

Report any side effects to doctor if severe or persistent. Those in orange, report immediately.

Important side effects	Negative drug interactions	Special warnings
colchicine, an antigout drug		$
Diarrhea, vomiting, nausea, stomach pain, rash, hives, swelling of face, lips, tongue, eyelids and throat, fever, fatigue, chills, sore throat, bruising, bleeding	**Do not combine with:** herbal teas. **Use caution with:** Biaxin (clarythromycin), erythromycin, and Sandimmune (cyclosporine).	**Do not use if:** you have an ulcer, ulcerative colitis; a kidney, liver, blood cell, or heart disorder; will have surgery in the near future; or have had a recent head injury. If you have asthma, chronic bronchitis, or emphysema, *colchicine* could cause respiratory difficulty. **Use caution if:** you have peptic ulcer disease or will have surgery in the near future. Discontinue if nausea occurs.
Zyloprim (allopurinol), an antigout drug		$
Rash, drowsiness, nausea, diarrhea, blood or bone marrow disorders that may produce fatigue, bleeding, or bruising, yellow eyes or skin, severe skin reactions marked by rashes, skin ulcers, hives, and itching, chest tightness, weakness	**Do not combine with:** aspirin, Capoten (captopril), Imuran (azathioprine), Vasotec (enalapril), iron or thiazide diuretics. **Use caution with:** Anturane (sulfinpyrazone), cyclosporine, probenecid, Purinethol (mercaptopurine), theophylline, and vitamin C.	**Do not use if:** you are having an acute gout attack. **Use caution if:** you have a history of hemochromatosis; have liver or kidney disease, epilepsy, or a blood cell or bone marrow disorder. Excessive vitamin C can increase risk of kidney stones. A low protein diet may increase side effects.

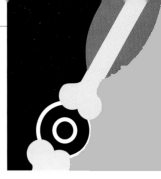

Osteoporosis

Symptoms: complications include compression, severe backache, hip, wrist and spine fractures.

Common drugs for osteoporosis

Report any side effects to doctor if severe or persistent. Those in orange, report immediately.

Important side effects	Negative drug interactions	Special warnings
Estrace *(estradiol)*, female sex hormone		$
Premarin *(conjugated estrogens)*, female sex hormone		$
Prempro *(conjugated estrogens)*, female sex hormone		$$

Abdominal bloating, stomach cramps, appetite loss, breast tenderness, breakthrough bleeding, nausea, vomiting, diarrhea, breast pain or enlargement, swelling of legs and feet, rapid weight gain, sudden or severe headache, loss of coordination, vision changes, pain in chest, groin or leg, shortness of breath, slurred speech, weakness or numbness in arm or leg	*Use caution with:* anticoagulants *(dicumarol, Miradon, warfarin),* anticonvulsants (Depakene, Dilantin, Tegretol), barbiturates (Amytal, Seconal, *phenobarbital),* Dantrium *(dantrolene),* major tranquilizers, oral antidiabetics (Amaryl, Glucotrol, Micronase), Rifadin *(rifampin),* steroids, thyroid preparations, tricyclic antidepressants (Aventyl, Elavil, Vivactil), and vitamin C.	*Do not use if:* you have liver problems, abnormal vaginal bleeding, sickle cell disease, breast cancer, estrogen-dependent cancer, or a history of thrombophlebitis, embolism, heart attack, or stroke. *Use caution if:* you have had a bad reaction to estrogen therapy; a history of breast or reproductive organ cancer or blood-clotting disorders; or have fibrocystic breast changes, fibroid tumors of the uterus, endometriosis, migraine-like headaches, epilepsy, asthma, heart disease, high blood pressure, gallbladder disease, diabetes, or porphyria; or if you will have surgery in the near future.

Evista *(raloxifene)*, a selective estrogen receptor modulator $$$$

Abdominal pain, arthritis, breast pain, chest pain, depression, fever, flu symptoms, gas, gynecological problems, hot flashes, coughing, indigestion, infection, swelling of throat and sinus passages, insomnia, joint pain, leg cramps, muscle aches, nausea, rash, sweating, swelling, urinary tract infection, vomiting, weight gain	*Use caution with:* Atromid-S *(clofibrate),* Coumadin *(warfarin),* estrogen, *ibuprofen,* Indocin *(indomethacin),* Naprosyn *(naproxen),* Questran *(cholestyramine),* and Valium *(diazepam).*	*Do not use if:* you have a history of blood clots or breast cancer. *Use caution if:* you have a history of thrombophlebitis or pulmonary embolism, impaired liver function, or a diet low in calcium or Vitamin D, or if you will have surgery in the near future. You should take calcium supplements while on this drug.

Common drugs for osteoporosis *continued*

Important side effects	Negative drug interactions	Special warnings

Fosamax *(alendronate)*, a bone resorption inhibitor $$$$

General pain, back pain, abdominal pain, bloating, indigestion, heartburn, nausea	*Do not combine with:* food, alcohol and Bufferin (aspirin). Take Fosamax only with water, never with food or coffee. Take a calcium supplement a half-hour after taking Fosamax. *Use caution with:* antacids, aspirin, and calcium supplements. Separate dosages of all other medications by at least 30 minutes.	*Do not use if:* kidney or esophageal disease or difficulty emptying the esophagus, or if you are unable to sit or stand for 30 minutes after taking each dose. *Use caution if:* you have ulcers or inflammation of the duodenum, difficulty swallowing, a calcium or Vitamin D deficiency, or depression. Stand-up or sit for 30 minutes after taking to keep drug from sitting in the stomach or esophagus, where it can cause irritation and ulceration.

Calcium carbonate with Vitamin D
Calcium citrate with Vitamin D

Constipation, diarrhea, black, tarry stools, or stools that look like coffee grounds	*Use caution with:* aspirin and other salicylates, magnesium-containing antacids, sodium polystyrene sulfonate, *quinidine,* and thiazide diuretics.	*Do not use if:* you have high blood levels of calcium. *Use caution if:* a history of heart or blood vessel disease, pancreatitis, or kidney problems. The Vitamin D increases absorption of the calcium, but too much can be toxic. You should have periodic tests to check levels of calcium, phosphorous, and Vitamin D. Separate doses of other drugs by 2 hours. Separate doses of quinolone antibiotics by 6 hours. Take after meals.

He said, she said, NSAIDs

Who said NSAIDs (pronounced **EN-SEDS**) were totally safe? If your doctor did, you may want to consider changing doctors. Non-steroidal anti-inflammatory drugs (known familiarly as NSAIDs) are effective in treating arthritis, but they come with a set of very serious warnings. They can cause serious, and sometimes fatal, reactions.

The group of drugs called NSAIDs include aspirin, ibuprofen, and the active ingredients in Aleve, Naprox, Voltaren, and Indocin. A study reported in the **New England Journal of Medicine** estimated that ulcers and ulcer-related complications caused by NSAIDs kill about 16,500 people in the U.S. each year.

Extreme caution is advised when combining NSAIDs with certain other drugs. For example, an NSAID combined with the anticoagulant drug Coumadin *(warfarin)*, could lead to bleeding ulcers. An NSAID combined with the anti-cancer drug Mexate *(methotrexate)* can lead to gastrointestinal problems, kidney failure, blood abnormalities, and in some cases, death.

The wise patient will use NSAIDs with extreme caution and always check with a doctor and a pharmacist before combining them with any other drug.

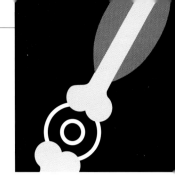

Osteoporosis

Osteoporosis, a condition that weakens bone, is largely a women's concern. It is estimated that in the U.S., at least 80% of sufferers are female. To understand the condition, it is helpful to start with the two basic bone cell types in our bodies. Osteoblasts, also known as bone formers, incorporate blood calcium and other minerals into bone. Osteoclasts dissolve bone and release calcium into the bloodstream.

When both of these cell types are functioning properly, they maintain a healthy balance. Bones are in continuous flux of building up and breaking down. It is when that balance is disrupted that osteoporosis sets in. Once a woman goes through menopause, her body stops producing estrogen. Estrogen is an important inhibitor of osteoclasts, so when it diminishes, osteoclasts are left free to dissolve bone faster than their partners the osteoblasts can replace it.

Calcimar, Estrace, Fosamax, and Premarin are all examples of osteoclast inhibitors that are used to take over where the natural estrogen left off.

Women at higher risk for osteoporosis are those who are small-boned, thin, and fair-haired, and women who smoke, drink more than moderately, or lead a sedentary lifestyle. Women who have a family history of osteoporosis are at higher risk, as are those who have had their ovaries removed, especially before the age of 40.

Epilepsy, too, is under intense scrutiny, as scientists search for a cause and cure. Meanwhile, new drugs inhibit or change brain cell activity to control seizures better.

There was a time when scientists believed the brain was too complicated to understand. Today, researchers believe cures for major brain disorders are possible. That's quite an advancement in itself.

Some things get better with age

Your likelihood of developing Alzheimer's climbs after age 60, peaks, but then starts to decline in your 70s, so if you make it to 85 without developing it, you have a lower risk than someone who is 65–70. Some 40% of people aged 85 have the disease.

Alzheimer's disease

Symptoms: memory loss and the inability to carry out daily activities. This doesn't mean forgetting where you left your car keys or to buy bread. It means seeing your car keys and not remembering what they are for or failing to recognize close family members.

 General Warnings

- **Do not stop these drugs abruptly. Sudden decline in thinking ability could occur.**
- **Do not use herbal medications for an extended period of time.**

Common drugs for Alzheimer's disease

Report any side effects to doctor if severe or persistent. Those in orange, report immediately.

Important side effects	Negative drug interactions	Special warnings
Aricept (donepezil), an acetylcholinesterase inhibitor		$$$$
Nausea, vomiting, diarrhea, headache, dizziness, fatigue, sleeping difficulty, changes in color of stools	Use caution with: anesthesia, antispasmodics, Decadron (dexamethasone), Dilantin (phenytoin), muscle relaxants, nonsteroidal anti-inflammatories, Nizoral (ketoconazole), Norvir (ritonavir), phenobarbital, Quinate (quinidine), Quinidex (quinidine), rifampin, Tegretol (carbamazepine), and Urecholine (bethanechol chloride).	Use caution if: you have a liver or seizure disorder, heart problems, low blood pressure, or glaucoma or a history of seizures or peptic ulcer disease. Do not stop these drugs abruptly.

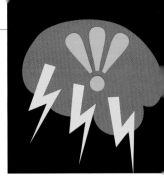

Common drugs for Alzheimer's disease *continued*		
Important side effects	**Negative drug interactions**	**Special warnings**
Tacrine, an antidementia agent		$$$$
Nausea, vomiting, stomach pain or cramps, indigestion, muscle aches or pains, headache, dizziness, appetite loss, diarrhea, clumsiness, unsteadiness, severe vomiting, rapid or pounding heartbeat, slow heartbeat, seizures, elevated liver function tests	*Use caution with:* antispasmodics, Artane *(trihexyphenidyl)*, Cogentin *(benztropine)*, Luvox *(fluvoxamine)*, muscle relaxants or stimulants, nonsteroidal anti-inflammatories (Aleve, Daypro, Toradol), Tagamet *(cimetidine)*, Theo-Dur *(theophylline)*, and Urecholine *(bethanechol chloride)*.	*Use caution if:* you have a liver or seizure disorder, heart problems, low blood pressure, or glaucoma or a history of seizures or peptic ulcer disease. Do not stop these drugs abruptly. Do not take with food.
Ginkgo biloba		
Spasms, cramps, mild digestive problems	*Use caution with:* antithrombotic therapy.	*Do not use if:* you are hypersensitive to Ginkgo biloba preparations. Acts as a blood thinner at higher doses.

Do you remember Dr. Alzheimer?

Near the beginning of the twentieth century, Dr. Alois Alzheimer conducted an autopsy on the brain of a woman who showed symptoms of senility for several years before dying in her mid-fifties. He discovered two main things: tangled nerve fibers and protein deposits dispersed over the cortex. Little did Dr. Alzheimer know at the time that he had made the first known diagnosis of Alzheimer's disease.

The 10 major warning signs or symptoms of Alzheimer's disease (AD)

- **Difficulty with familiar tasks.** The AD patient may walk out of a store without paying or even without buying half the items sought.

- **Slipping job performance.** AD patients may repeatedly go into a room and forget why, or fail to keep an appointment and forget it had ever been made.

- **Language difficulties.** People with AD may repeatedly forget common words or phrase words in an incomprehensible way.

- **Confusion of place and time.** AD patients may forget the year, get lost in their own homes, or fail to recognize loved ones.

- **Lack of judgment.** An AD patient may walk down a highway at midnight or put clothes on backwards.

- **Problems in abstract thinking.** People with AD may forget how to add numbers, or lose the ability to plan.

- **Misplacing objects.** An AD patient may place a book in the freezer or look for a pair of glasses in the sink.

- **Mood fluctuations.** A person with AD may laugh suddenly, then become angry, then sob uncontrollably.

- **Changes in personality.** An AD patient who was friendly and outgoing may become timid, shy, and suspicious.

- **Lack of initiative.** A person with AD may chew food and forget to swallow.

Parkinson's disease

Symptoms: weakness, tremor of head or hands, slow, jerky movements, shuffling gait, stooped posture, unsteadiness, difficulty rising from a sitting position, rubbing together of thumb and forefinger, indistinct speech, and swallowing problems.

Common drugs for Parkinson's disease

Report any side effects to doctor if severe or persistent. Those in orange, report immediately.

Important side effects	Negative drug interactions	Special warnings
Cogentin *(benztropine)*, an anti-Parkinson's drug		$
Constipation, heartbeat changes, abnormal behavior, confusion, bowel obstruction	***Do not combine with:*** antipsychotics (Haldol, Serentil, Thorazine) and tricyclic antidepressants (Aventyl, Elavil, Vivactil). ***Use caution with:*** alcohol, antihistamines, other anticholinergics, over-the-counter medications, Sinequan *(doxepin)*, and Symmetrel *(amantadine)*. Do not take antacids within one hour of taking benztropine.	***Do not use if:*** you have tardive dyskinesia or glaucoma. ***Use caution if:*** you have had a bad reaction to atropine-like drugs; have myasthenia gravis, heart disease, or high blood pressure; a history of liver or kidney disease; have bowel obstructions or difficulty urinating; have taken an MAO inhibitor in the last 14 days; or will soon be exposed to extreme heat.
Eldepryl *(selegiline)*, an anti-Parkinson's drug		$$
Nausea, dry mouth, dizziness, low blood pressure which causes lightheadedness, fainting and confusion, involuntary muscle movements, abnormal heartbeat	***Do not combine with:*** Demerol *(meperidine)*, Luvox *(fluvoxamine)*, Meridia *(sibutramine)*, phenylpropanolamine, Sudafed *(pseudoephedrine)*, Ultram *(tramadol)*, and Wellbutrin *(buproprion)*. ***Use caution with:*** alcohol, antidiabetics (Glucophage, Glucophage, Precose), Dexedrine *(amphetamine)*, dextromethorphan (a cough suppressant ingredient), Effexor *(venlafaxine)*, Humulin *(insulin)*, Lithobid *(lithium)*, Meridia *(sibutramine)*, Paxil *(paroxetine)*, Prozac *(fluoxetine)*, *tryptophan*, and Zoloft *(sertraline)*, antidepressants that raise serotonin levels (Paxil, Prozac, Zoloft), antihypertensives, antipsychotics (Clozaril, Haldol, Thorazine), *levodopa*, narcotic painkillers, and tricyclic antidepressants (Aventyl, Elavil, Vivactil).	***Do not use if:*** you have Huntington's disease, hereditary tremor, or tardive dyskinesia (a nervous disorder with involuntary movements of eyelids, jaws, lips, tongue, neck and fingers). ***Use caution if:*** you have low blood pressure, peptic ulcer disease, or a history of heart rhythm disorder.

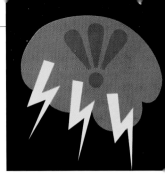

Common drugs for Parkinson's disease *continued*

Important side effects	Negative drug interactions	Special warnings

Permax *(pergolide)*, an anti-Parkinson's drug $$$$

Dizziness or lightheadedness when standing or sitting up suddenly, confusion, hallucinations, unusual or abnormal muscle movements, low blood pressure which causes dizziness, lightheadedness, fainting and confusion, painful urination	*Use caution with:* alcohol, antihypertensives (Hytrin, Cardura, Catapres), antipsychotics (Clozaril, Haldol, Thorazine).	*Do not use if:* you have had an adverse reaction to an ergot preparation or have coronary artery disease or peripheral vascular disease. *Use caution if:* you have low blood pressure, a heart or seizure disorder, or impaired liver or kidney function.

Sinemet, anti-Parkinson's drug $
Dopar *(levodopa)*, anti-Parkinson's drug $$$$$

Nausea, confusion, involuntary muscle movements, irregular heartbeat, low blood pressure, fainting or near fainting, hallucinations, fatigue, depression, dizziness, light-headedness when standing or sitting up suddenly	*Do not combine with:* Catapres *(clonidine),* INH *(isoniazid),* MAO inhibitor antidepressants (Marplan, Nardil, Parnate), phenothiazines (Compazine, Permitil, Serentil), and Risperdal *(risperidone).* *Use caution with:* antacids, anticonvulsants (Depakene, Dilantin, Tegretol), antihypertensives, antispasmodics, high protein foods, iron, MAO inhibitors (Marplan, Nardil, Parnate), major tranquilizers, Nydrazid *(isoniazid),* Pavabid *(papaverine),* Reglan *(metoclopramide),* tranquilizers, and Vitamin B6 *(pyridoxine).* Consult your doctor before combining these drugs with any other drug. They interact with many other medications.	*Do not use if:* you have glaucoma or a history of melanoma or if you have taken an MAO inhibitor in the last 14 days. *Use caution if:* you have diabetes, epilepsy, heart disease, high blood pressure, chronic lung disease; liver, kidney, or heart disorders; a history of mental illness, peptic ulcer disease, or malignant melanoma. Do not take these drugs with protein foods.

Symmetrel *(amantadine)*, an antiviral and anti-Parkinson's drug $

Dizziness, irritability, distractability, difficulty sleeping, rash, confusion, seizures, hallucinations, swollen feet or arms, difficulty breathing, shortness of breath on exertion or at night, cough, swelling of feet or ankles	*Do not combine with:* alcohol, Artane *(trihexyphenidyl),* Cogentin *(benztropine).* *Use caution with:* amphetamines, cotrimoxazole, Dyazide (hydrochlorothiazide), *levodopa, sulfamethoxazole,* and *trimethoprim.*	*Use caution if:* you have a seizure disorder, liver or kidney problems, eczema or eczema-like rashes, or a history of mental disorders, heart problems, lowered blood pressure upon standing, peptic ulcer disease, or low white blood cell counts. Avoid exposure to anyone with German measles.

> Very few people go to the doctor when they have a cold. They go to the theater instead.
>
> W. BOYD GATEWOOD
> *quoted in* Reader's Digest
> *June 1949*

Asthma

Symptoms: shortness of breath, wheezing that may begin as a slight whistling sound, coughing that gets worse over minutes or hours, faster breathing, blue nails and lips, sudden anxiety and apprehension, swelling of the mucous lining of the airways within the lungs, and excessive production of a thick mucus.

STOP General Warnings

- Call your doctor if you develop a skin rash or hives while taking any of the following drugs.
- Do not use herbal medications for an extended period of time.

Common drugs for asthma

Report any side effects to doctor if severe or persistent. Those in orange, report immediately.

Important side effects	Negative drug interactions	Special warnings
Accolate *(zafirlukast)*, leukotriene receptor antagonist		$$$
Singulair *(montelukast)*, leukotriene receptor antagonist		$$$
Zyflo *(zileuton)*, leukotriene receptor antagonist		$$$
Headache, stomach upset, flu-like symptoms, increased number of infections, burning or prickling sensation, rash	*Do not use with:* theophylline. *Use caution with:* aspirin, beta blockers (Inderal, Tenormin, Toprol), calcium channel blockers (Adalat CC, Cardizem, Norvasc), Coumadin *(warfarin),* cyclosporine, Dilantin *(phenytoin),* erythromycin, Hismanal *(astemizole),* Orinase *(tolbutamide),* Tegretol *(carbamazepine),* and Theo-Dur *(theophylline).*	*Do not use if:* you have liver disease or increased liver enzymes. Do not take with food. *Use caution if:* you have an acute asthma attack, impaired kidney function, or drink a lot of alcohol. Liver function tests may be necessary.

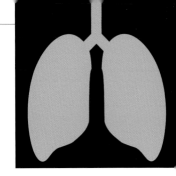

Common drugs for asthma *continued*

Important side effects	Negative drug interactions	Special warnings
Azmacort *(triamcinolone)*, corticosteroid		$$$
AeroBid *(flunisolide)*, corticosteroid		$$$$
Beclovent *(beclomethasone)*, corticosteroid		$$$$
Decadron *(dexamethasone)*, corticosteroid		$
Flovent *(fluticasone)*, corticosteroid		$$$$
Pulmicort *(budesonide)*, corticosteroid		$$$$$
Vanceril *(beclomethasone)*, corticosteroid		$$$
Irritation of the mouth, tongue and throat, fungal infections in mouth, voice changes	*Use caution with:* digoxin, insulin, oral antidiabetics (Amaryl, Glucophage, Glucotrol), and Coumadin (warfarin).	*Do not use if:* you need to treat symptoms quickly or if you have a fungal infection. *Use caution if:* you have ever taken a cortisone-related drug; have a history of tuberculosis; or have chronic bronchitis or bronchiectasis, diabetes, glaucoma, myasthenia gravis, peptic ulcer disease, hypothyroidism, or an infection. Call your doctor if severe asthma returns while you are taking Azmacort. Watch for signs of lung infection. Rinse mouth after use to minimize side effects.
Proventil *(albuterol)*, bronchodilator/sympathomimetic		$
Ventolin *(albuterol)*, bronchodilator/sympathomimetic		$
Nervousness, tremor, dizziness, headache, insomnia, chest pain or heaviness, irregular heartbeat, lightheadedness, fainting, weakness, headache	*Use caution with:* antidepressants (Elavil, Nardil, Prozac), beta blockers (Inderal, Sectral, Tenormin), digitalis, Lanoxin (digoxin), drugs similar to albuterol, drugs that lower potassium levels, and stimulants.	*Do not use if:* you have an irregular heart rhythm or hyperthyroidism, or have taken an MAO inhibitor in the last 14 days. *Use caution if:* you have a heart or circulatory disorder or diabetes. Do not take albuterol until at least two weeks after your last dose of an MAOI antidepressant. Do not use albuterol excessively. Avoid excessive caffeine.

Bronchitis

Symptoms: a hacking cough, yellow or green phlegm, fever, chills, soreness and tightness in chest, pain below breastbone during deep breathing.

Common drugs for acute bronchitis

Report any side effects to doctor if severe or persistent. Those in orange, report immediately.

Important side effects	Negative drug interactions	Special warnings
ampicillin—see sinusitis		
amoxicillin—see sinusitis		
Bactrim DS *(sulfamethoxazole)*, see urinary tract infection		
Biaxin *(clarithromycin)*, see sinusitis		
Ery-Tab *(erythromycin)*, a macrolide antibiotic		$
Stomach cramps, abdominal discomfort, diarrhea, nausea, vomiting, fever, nausea, skin reddening or itching, severe stomach pain, yellow eyes or skin, fainting, slow or irregular heartbeat, breathing difficulty, persistent or severe diarrhea, abdominal pain, temporary deafness	*Do not combine with:* alcohol. *Use with caution with:* anticonvulsants (Depakene, Dilantin, Tegretol), Cafergot *(ergotamine)*, Coumadin *(warfarin)*, cyclosporine, dihydroergotamine, Halcion *(triazolam)*, Lanoxin *(digoxin)*, Mevacor *(lovastatin)*, Norpace *(disopyramide)*, Parlodel *(bromocriptine)*, Prograf *(tacrolimus)*, Tegretol *(carbamazepine)*, and Theo-Dur *(theophylline)*.	*Do not use if:* you have liver disease or are allergic to para-amniobenzoic-acid-type anesthetics. *Use caution if:* you have had a bad reaction to macrolide antibiotics; have allergies, a blood disorder, abnormal heart rhythm, myasthenia gravis, or a hearing disorder; have a history of porphyria, liver or kidney disorder, or low blood platelets; or have previously taken the estolate form of *erythromycin*. Do not drink fruit juices and carbonated beverages for at least one hour after taking *erythromycin*.
Levaquin *(levofloxacin)*, a fluoroquinolone antibiotic		?????
Increased sensitivity to sunlight, seizures, mental confusion, hallucinations, agitation, nightmares, depression, shortness of breath, unusual swelling in face or extremities, loss of conciousness, increased risk of tendinitis or tendon rupture, mental changes	*Use caution with:* Coumadin *(warfarin)*, nonsteroidal anti-inflammatories (Aleve, Daypro, Toradol), oral antidiabetics (Amaryl, Glucotrol, Micronase), *probenecid*, other quinolone antibiotics, and *theophylline*.	*Do not use if:* you have a seizure disorder or "long Q-T syndrome" (a rare genetic disorder). *Use caution if:* you are allergic to quinolone antibiotics, (Cipro, Floxin), or if you have a brain circulatory disorder, impaired liver or kidney function, a history of mental illness, or if you do heavy manual labor. Drink a lot of water while taking Levaquin.

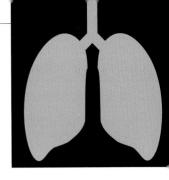

Common drugs for acute bronchitis *continued*		
Important side effects	**Negative drug interactions**	**Special warnings**
Echinacea		
		Do not use if: you have AIDS, autoimmune diseases such as rheumatoid arthritis and lupus, leukemia, leukoses, collagenoses, tuberculosis, or multiple sclerosis. Parenteral administration should not be given to people with allergies.
Thyme		
Wild Cherry		

Sinusitis

Symptoms: nasal congestion and thick discharge, fever, chills, frontal headache, and painful swelling in the sinuses.

Common drugs for sinusitis		
Report any side effects to doctor if severe or persistent. Those in orange, report immediately.		
Important side effects	**Negative drug interactions**	**Special warnings**
***amoxicillin*, penicillin antibiotic**		$
***ampicillin*, penicillin antibiotic**		$
Rash, diarrhea, nausea, vomiting, headache, vaginal discharge and itching, pain or white patches in mouth or on tongue, irregular breathing, lightheadedness, sudden fainting, joint pain, fever, severe abdominal pain and cramping with watery or bloody stools, sudden swelling of lips, tongue, face or throat, breathing difficulty, rash, itching, hives, unusual bleeding or bruising, yellow eyes or skin	***Use caution with:*** Aralen *(chloroquine)*, Benemid *(probenecid)*, Chloromycetin *(chloramphenicol)*, Coumadin *(warfarin)*, Lariam *(mefloquine)*, Mexate *(methotrexate)*, oral contraceptives (Loestrin, Nordette, Ortho Cyclen), Tenormin *(atenolol)*, and Zyloprim *(allopurinol)*.	***Do not use if:*** you are allergic to penicillin. ***Use caution if:*** you are allergic to any cephalosporin antibiotic, or if you have allergies, or a history of liver or kidney disease or low blood counts.

Common drugs for sinusitis *continued*

Important side effects	Negative drug interactions	Special warnings

Biaxin *(clarithromycin)*, a macrolide antibiotic $$$

Colitis (with symptoms including severe abdominal pain or cramping, watery or bloody stools, severe diarrhea, fever), nausea, vomiting, yellow eyes or skin, swelling of lips, tongue, face and throat, breathing difficulty, rash, hives, unusual bleeding, bruising, red spots on skin, confusion, changes in behavior, heartbeat irregularities	**Do not combine with:** ergot alkaloids, Gerimal *(ergoloid mesylates)*, and Valium *(diazepam)*. **Use caution with:** Betapace *(soltalol)*, BuSpar *(buspirone)*, Cafergot *(ergotamine)*, Codarone *(amiodarone)*, Coumadin *(warfarin)*, cyclosporine, Depakote *(valporic acid)*, Diflucan *(fluconazole)*, Dilantin *(phenytoin)*, Halcion *(triazolam)*, Lanoxin *(digoxin)*, Lithobid *(lithium)*, Mexate *(trimexate)*, Mevacor *(lovastatin)*, midazolam, Norpace *(disopyramide)*, Norvir *(ritonavir)*, Orap *(pimozide)*, Parlodel *(bromocriptine)*, phenothiazines (Compazine, Permitil, Trilafon), Prograf *(tacrolimus)*, Propulsid *(cisapride)*, quinolone antibiotics, Retrovir *(zidovudine)*, Rifadin *(rifampin)*, Seldane *(terfenadine)*, Tegretol *(carbamazepine)*, theophylline, valporate, Viagra *(sildenafil)*, and Viramune *(nevirapine)*.	**Use caution if:** you have had a bad reation to a macrolide antibiotic; have allergies, a blood disorder, abnormal heart rhythm, myasthenia gravis, or a hearing disorder; have a history of porphyria, kidney disorders, or low blood platelets; or have taken the estolate form of erythromycin previously.

Lorabid *(loracarbef)*, a cephalosporin antibiotic $$$$

Appetite loss, diarrhea, stomach pain, nausea, vomiting, severe diarrhea, rash, hives, itching	**Use caution with:** Diuretics and Benemid *(probenecid)*.	**Do not use if:** you are allergic to any cephalosporin. **Use caution if:** you have a history of allergy to penicillin, or if you have impaired kidney function, or a history of regional enteritis, ulcerative colitis, blood clotting disorders, low platelets, or white blood cell counts.

Zithromax *(azithromycin)*, a macrolide antibiotic $$

Breathing difficulty, fever, hives, itching, rash, swelling of face, mouth, lips, throat or tongue, sweating, yellow eyes or skin	**Use caution with:** antacids containing aluminum or magnesium, antihistamines, Coumadin *(warfarin)*, Crixivan *(indinavir)*, cyclosporine, digoxin, Dilantin *(phenytoin)*, ergot-containing drugs, Halcion *(triazolam)*, Mevacor	**Do not use if:** you have had a bad reaction to a macrolide antibiotic **Use caution if:** you have allergies, a blood disorder, abnormal heart rhythm, myasthenia gravis, or a hearing disorder; a history of porphyria,

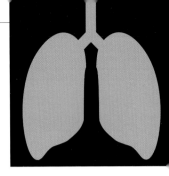

Common drugs for sinusitis *continued*		
Important side effects	**Negative drug interactions**	**Special warnings**
Zithromax *continued*		
	(lovastatin), Sporanox *(itra-conazole),* Tegretol *(carba-mazepine),* and *theophylline.*	kidney disorders, or low blood platelets; or have taken the estolate form of *erythromycin* previously.
Advil Cold and Sinus *(pseudoephedrine)*		
Bayer Select Aspirin-Free Sinus Pain Relief *(pseudoephedrine)*		
Excedrin Sinus *(pseudoephedrine)*		
Nervousness, restlessness, excitability, insomnia, dizziness, weakness, headache, drowsiness	*Do not combine with:* MAO inhibitor antidepressants (Marplan, Nardate, Parnate). Use caution when combining these drugs with caffeine and other decongestants (Allerest, Dristan 12-Hour, Sinarest).	*Use caution if:* you have hyperthyroidism, heart disease, high blood pressure, diabetes, or an enlarged prostate. Do not take for more than seven consecutive days, unless directed by your doctor. Do not take within two weeks of stopping an MAO inhibitor antidepressant.

What do you take for a cold?

Have you ever walked down the cold medicine aisle at your local pharmacy? The number of choices is overwhelming when you're feeling well and downright mind-boggling when you've got a pounding headache, a stuffy nose, watery eyes and a sore throat.

Fortunately, there's a simple solution. An advisory panel to the Food and Drug Administration has recommended that if you are going to take something for a cold, it should be a single-ingredient medicine. The problem with multiple-ingredient medicines is that they will cause more side effects and may make you feel worse. Also many over-the-counter drugs interact with food and prescription medications. So, decide which of your symptoms is the worst and treat it alone. Ask your pharmacist for recommendations. As your cold progresses, so too will your symptoms, so you should adapt your treatment strategy accordingly.

Active ingredients in cold medicines are those that attack your symptoms. They are **analgesics** (painkillers), **antipyretics** (fever reducers), **decongestants** (which relieve stuffy noses and sinuses), **cough suppressants,** and **expectorants** (which liquefy and loosen phlegm so it will be coughed up). Some antihistamines (which counter the symptoms of allergies) are also used in cold medications—not because of their effect on allergies but because they cause nasal drying.

A Symptom Translation List

Agranulocytosis
An acute feverish condition marked by severe decrease in blood granulocytes

Akathisia
Restless leg syndrome

Akinesia
Weakness, muscle fatigue

Amblyopia
Dimmed sight, especially in one eye

Anuria
Diminished or absence of urine output

Aphasia
Inability to speak or understand words

Aplastic/hypoplastic anemia
Anemia that is characterized by defective function of the blood-forming organs

Arthralgia
Pain in one or more joints

Asthenia
Loss of body strength, weakness

Ataxia
Inability to coordinate voluntary body movements

Bradycardia
Abnormally slow heartbeat

Dyspnea
Difficult breathing

Glomerulonephritis
A type of kidney infection

Glycosuria
Sugar in the urine

Hyperuricemia
Excess uric acid in the blood

Lactic acidosis
A build-up of lactic acid in the blood that is often fatal

Leukocytosis
Increased white blood cells in the circulating blood

Lymphadenopathy
Enlarged lymph nodes

Myalgia
Muscle pain

Nocturia
A need to urinate at night that disturbs sleep

Paresthesia
A prickling, creeping, or tickling sensation in the skin

Pericardial effusion
Fluid buildup in the pericardium, a sac around the heart

Polyuria
Excessive urination

Pruritus
Intense itching

Purpura
Purple patches of skin

Sjogren's syndrome
Marked by swollen glands, dry mouth/eyes, and arthritis

Splenomegaly
Enlargement of the spleen

Tachycardia
Racing heart

Tardive dyskinesia
Lip smacking, tongue rolling, other involuntary movements

Thrombocytopenia
Decreased blood platelet count, usually from hemorrhaging

Urticaria
Itchy rash, hives

Vertigo
Dizziness

Xanthopsia
Yellow vision

TOP Hit List

The diseases generating "the greatest use of the Web" were depression (19%), cancer (15%), bipolar disorder (14%) and arthritis or rheumatism (10%), according to a 1999 Harris poll.

Online Resources

Last year, about 22 million people went looking for health information on the Internet, according to **Cyber Dialog Inc.**, an Internet market research firm in New York. Estimates predict the figure will grow to 33 million by the end of 2000. Of those, about 70% did health research before going to their doctors' offices. And, although only 20 percent of older adult have access to the Internet, the 50-plus set represents the fastest growing segment on the online community.

Here's what you can do online:

- Consult with a doctor. **AmericasDoctor.com** offers private consultation with online docs— for free. For $195, **Mediconsult.com** will send you a report on your health history, analyze test results, and offer treatment options, but not make diagnoses or prescribe medicine. **CyberDocs.com** offers virtual doctors appointments. You exchange information. The site is intended for minor medical problems and costs between $50 to $75 per appointment.

- Fill a prescription.

  drugstore.com

  planetrx.com

  cvs.com

- Research medical information. Some of the top sites are:

  nih.gov/health

  onhealth.com

  intelihealth.com

  pharminfo.com

  healthcentral.com

  mayo.edu

- Find clinical trials.

  MedTrial.com

  drkoop.com

  clinicaltrials.com

  CenterWatch.com

  nci.hih.gov
  (*National Cancer Institute*)

- Chat with other patients who share your concerns.

- Store your health records. At **PersonalMD.com**, you can set up your own personalized health home page, keep history, emergency contacts, x-ray and EKG reports.

Clearly, the Internet a rich source of information, but misinformation abounds as well and cyber-savvy hucksters who will promise to cure you of all your problems.

Weeding out questionable online information
Operation Cure

The **Federal Trade Commission** launched **Operation Cure**. All to police websites and team with **Health and Human Services** to run consumer education campaigns aimed at helping consumers distinguish good Web sites from bad ones.

The **U.S. Office of Consumer Affairs** lists product statements that should alert consumers to be skeptical. Here are some red flags:

- Products touted as miracle drugs, revolutionary breakthroughs, or magic bullets and are available only from one source.

- Claims that the product is quick, painless, and effortless—and will cure a wide range of diseases.

- Products purported to have secret, foreign, or ancient ingredients.

- Promoters claim doctors don't want you to know about this product or they refuse to acknowledge its effectiveness.

- Claims of effectiveness based on personal stories rather than scientific research or based on a single study without peer review.

Complementary medicine:

For adverse effects from herbs. You can find adverse effects reported to **FDA** at this website **vm.cfsan.fda.gov/~dms/aems.html** (call the FDA Hotline at **800.332.1088** to report adverse events)

American Botanical Council for information on the safe use of drugs
www.herbalgram.org

National Institute of Health's National Centre for Complementary and Alternative Medicine nccam.nih.gov/nccam/what-is-cam/

Alternative and Complementary Medicine Center allows you to search for practitioners **www.healthy.net/clinic/therapy/index.asp**

The **Office of Alternative Medicine** sponsored by the U.S. Government gives research information on alternative therapies
scrdp.standord.edu/camps.html

Holistic Internet Resource
www.healthy.net

Website Bookmarks Used For This Book

Here are the sites used to research this book. Those with a red dot were particularly useful:

www.usp.org

aaom.org

accenthealth.com

- agenet.com

altimed.com

altmedicine.com

ama-assn.org/aps/amahg.htm

americangeriatrics.org

ascp.com

cdc.gov/nchs

centerwatch.com

chronicillnet.org

citizen.org

cvs.com

docboard.org

drugawareness.org

drugdigest.org

eldercare.com

elderweb.com/drugs.htm

- EL.com/elinks/medicine
Essential Links to Medicine

excite.com/health/alternative_medicine

fda.gov/cder/adr

fda.gov/cder/consumerinfo

fda.gov/cder/warn

fda.gov/fdac/special/newdrug/benefits.html

fda.gov/fdac/special/newdrug/ndd_toc.html

fda.gov/medwatch

health.org/pubs/elderly

- HealthAtoZ.com

health-center.com

healthcentral.com

healthfinder.gov

healthgate.com

healthtouch.com

healthy.net

himss.org
Healthcare Information Management
Systems Society

ihpr.ubc.ca/medicallinks.htm

imshealth.com

- intelihealth.com
Johns Hopkins

intmed.mcw.edu/drug.html

- mayo.edu

medicinenet.com

medinfo.org

- medscape.com

medsite.com

merck.com

mmhc.com/cg

multum.com

ncbi.nlm.nih.gov

nccam.nih.gov

nci.nih.gov

nci.nih.gov/atlas/mortality.html

nih.gov/health

nih.gov:80/nia

- nlm.nih.gov/medlineplus
National Library of Medicine

- nim.nih.gov/medlineplus/druginformation.html
FDA drug information in layman's terms

noah.cuny.edu/qksearch.html

onhealth.com

- pdr.net
Physician's Desk Reference

- pharminfo.com

powernetdesign.com/grapefruit

- rxlist.com

seniorliving.about.com/people/seniorliving

sick.com

springnet.com/ce/j609a.htm

- thriveonline.com

unitedhealthcare.com

wellweb.com/SENIORS/ELDERSHP.HTM

who.int
World Health Organization

Medical Organizations and Associations for Older Adults

American Geriatrics Society
770 Lexington Avenue, Suite 300
New York, NY 10021
212.308.1414
americangeriatrics.org

American Association of Retired Persons (AARP)
601 E. Street, NW
Washington, DC 20049
202.434.2277
aarp.org

American Society on Aging
833 Market Street, Suite 511
San Francisco, CA 94103
415.974.9600
asaging.org

American Society of Consultant Pharmacists
1321 Duke Street
Alexandria, VA 22314-3516
703.739.1300
ascp.com

Gerontological Society of America
1030 15th Street, NW, Suite 250
Washington, DC 20005
202.842.1275
geron.org

National Alliance for Senior Citizens
1744 Riggs Place, NW
Washington, DC 20009
202.986.0117
members.aol.com/nascfdn

National Council on the Aging
409 3rd Street, SW, Suite 200
Washington, DC 20024
202.479.1200
Ncoa.org

National Council on Patient Information and Education
666 11th Street, NW, Suite 810
Washington, DC 20001
202.347.6711
E-mail: ncpie@erols.com

National Health Information Center
POB 1133
Washington, DC 20013-1133
301.565.4167
nhic-nt.health.org

National Institute on Aging
Public Information Office
31 Center Drive, Room 5C27
Bethesda, MD 20892-2292
301.496.1752
nih.gov/nia

Index

Nitrostat, 59

nizatidine, 42

non-steroidal anti-inflammatory drugs, 100, 106

norfloxacin, 35

Noroxin, 35

Norpace, 55

Norvasc, 34, 59,67, 69

NSAIDs, 100, 106

nutraceuticals, 6

ofloxacin, 80

olsalazine, 40

omeprazole, 42

onion, 69

osteoporosis, 105, 107

oxaprozin, 100

oxybutynin chloride, 76

Parkinson's Disease, 112

Parnate, 35

paroxetine, 85, 89

parsley, 80

passion flower, 94

Paxil, 85, 89

penicillin, 35, 119

Pepcid, 42

peptic ulcer, 42

Pepto-Bismol, 43

pergolide, 113

Permax, 113

pharmacist, 13

phenobarbital, 35

pill planner, 9

pill profile, 8

pioglitazone, 46

Plavix, 70

Plendil, 34, 67

poke root, 24

potassium chloride, 62

potassium supplement, 62

potassium-sparing diuretic, 68

Pravachol, 64

pravastatin, 64

Prednisone, 100

Premarin, 50

Prempro, 50

Prevacid, 42

Prilosec, 42

primidone, 35

Prinivil, 60, 66, 69

procainamide, 55

Procan, 55

Procardia XL, 34, 59, 69

Proscar, 78

ProSom, 93

Prostate problems, 77

Proventil, 117

Provera, 49

Prozac, 85, 89

pseudoe phedrine, 121

psychotherapeutic, 111

Psyllium, 65

Pulmicort, 117

pumpkin seed, 78

Pygeum, 78

quazepam, 92

quinapril, 60, 66, 69

Quinidex, 56

quinidine, 56

raloxifene, 105

ramipril, 60, 66

reactions, 26

Relafen, 101

Restoril, 93

rofecoxib, 99

Rolaids, 43

rosiglitazone, 46

s-adenosyl-methionine, 91

SAMe, 91

sassafras, 24

Saw Palmetto, 78

Sectral, 56

Sectral, 68

seizures, 31

selective estrogen receptor modulator, 105

selective serotonin re-uptake inhibitor, 85

selegiline, 112

Septra, 79

sertraline, 85, 90

Serzone, 90

side effects, 21, 26, 28, 36, 37

sildenafil citrate, 74

simvastatin, 65

Sinemet, 113

Singulair, 116

sinusitis, 119

sleep disorders, 92

slippery elm, 41, 43

Slo-bid, 35

Slow-K, 62

sodium bicarbonate, 43

Sominex, 93

soy lectin, 65

Our Thanks

Loring Leifer for her tremendous efforts in research and writing.

Joel Katz, Dave Schpok, Jennifer Long, Mary Torrieri and Kerry Morozin at **Joel Katz Design Associates**, Philadelphia, PA for their design and production talents.

Ann Morris for her assistance with much of the research.

Paul Temme, Richard Routman and **Milton Ziman** for useful suggestions and wise counsel.

The following distinguished members of the medical and scientific community have been most generous with their time, their knowledge, and their insights. To each, we say thank you.

Dean Goldberg, Pharm.D., Vice President of Clinical Pharmacy Management, **UnitedHealthcare**, Minneapolis, MN

Linda Holliday, President, and **Michael Golub M.D., F.A.C.P.**, Vice President, Science and Medicine, **Medical Broadcasting Company**, Philadelphia, PA

Thelda Kestenbaum, M.D., Kansas University Medical Center, Kansas City, KS

Bill Leifer, M.D., Medical Director of Clinical Laboratories, **St. Francis Hospital and Medical Center**, Topeka, KS

John Mach, M.D., Chief Medical Officer, **EverCare**, Minneapolis, MN

Sharon Marx, M.D., Assistant Medical Director, **EverCare**, Minneapolis, MN

Allen Shaughnessey, Pharm.D., Director of Research, **Pinnacle Health/Harrisburg Family Practice Residency Program**, Harrisburg, PA

UMKC School of Pharmacy Drug Information Center, Kansas City, MO

Randall Wright, R.Ph., RJ Wright Consulting, Lake Lotawana, MO